SURGERY - PROCEDURES, COMPLICATIONS, AND RESULTS

THYROIDECTOMY

SURGICAL PROCEDURES, POTENTIAL COMPLICATIONS AND POSTOPERATIVE OUTCOMES

SURGERY - PROCEDURES, COMPLICATIONS, AND RESULTS

Additional books in this series can be found on Nova's website under the Series tab.

Additional e-books in this series can be found on Nova's website under the e-book tab.

SURGERY - PROCEDURES, COMPLICATIONS, AND RESULTS

THYROIDECTOMY

SURGICAL PROCEDURES, POTENTIAL COMPLICATIONS AND POSTOPERATIVE OUTCOMES

KIMBERLY RODOLFO
EDITOR

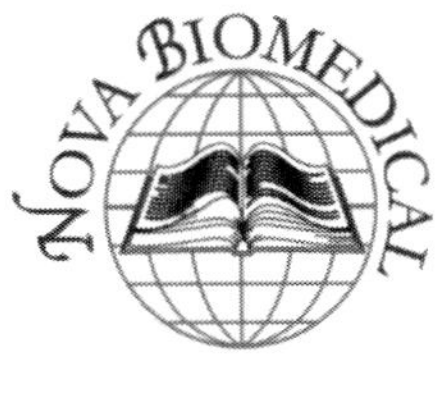

New York

For permission to use material from this book please contact us:
Telephone 631-231-7269; Fax 631-231-8175
Web Site: http://www.novapublishers.com

Library of Congress Cataloging-in-Publication Data

ISBN: 978-1-63321-440-8

Library of Congress Control Number: 2014943362

Published by Nova Science Publishers, Inc. † New York

Contents

Preface

The thyroid gland is located in the neck deep to the platysma. This is a broad sheet of muscle that crosses over the clavicle to cover the antero-lateral neck. Its anterior fibres interlace with the opposite side, finding an attachment to the mandible and the dermis of the lower part of the face. The platymsa covers the sternocleidomastoid and the strap muscles of the neck: sternothyroid, sternohyoid and omohyoid. In order to maximize aesthetics after thyroidectomy, surgeons use a transverse collar incision through the skin and platysma. This book discusses the surgical procedures taken during a thyroidectomy, and also explores the potential complications involved. Postoperative outcomes are also discussed.

Chapter 1 – The immunopathogenesis of Graves' disease (GD) is an evolving story, but the central role of Thyrotrophin receptor antibodies (TRAb) in its aetiology is well established. TRAb are primarily produced in intrathyroidal immune competent cells. In treatment naïve subjects, they are found as stimulating (TSAb), blocking (TBAb) or possible neutral TRAb. The clinical phenotype is therefore dependent on the dominant form in the blood i.e. GD when TSAb, and hypothyroidism when TBAb predominates. But currently commercially available assays in clinical use cannot differentiate between TSAb and TBAb and there is no consensus about the utility of TRAb, in diagnosing or predicting outcome in GD.

There are two assay types used to measure TRAb – "receptor assays" and "bioassays". Although these assays can detect TRAb in up to 95% of GD patients, only the currently relatively cumbersome, time consuming and more expensive bioassay can determine their functional characteristics. Their clinical utility is therefore limited to research. The more user friendly, easy to perform and cheaper receptor assays measure both TSAb and TBAb, and cannot differentiate between them. Therefore TRAb positivity in these assays does not predict clinical phenotype or outcome. Complicating these analytical imperfections, TRAb also has the ability to change from one type to the other during the course of the disease and its treatment. The clinician therefore has only an imperfect tool to diagnose and predict GD outcome.

TRAb measurement in clinical situations other than isolated GD, merits discussion - (a) GD complicates pregnancy in a minority and the utility of maternal TRAb measurement to predict foetal and neonatal problems due to tranpslacental TRAb transfer is well established. (b) The recently described "Immune reconstitution syndrome" in patients receiving drugs such as Alemtuzumab and the highly active anti retrovirals (HAART), predisposes affected individuals to GD, and TRAb assays help diagnosis. (c) The occurrence of typical Graves' orbitopathy (GO) in hypothyroid and euthyroid patients and (d) unilateral GO are also situations where TRAb measurement helps.

Chapter 2 – Albrecht von Haller first described an Intra-Thoracic Goiter (ITG) in 1749. Terms such as retrosternal, sub-sternal, intrathoracic, or mediastinal have also been used to define a goiter that extends beyond the thoracic inlet. Incidence in the general population, based on mass chest Computed Tomography (CT) screening, is 0.02 – 0.5%. The diagnosis of ITG is frequently made in the fifth or sixth decade of life, with a male/female rate of 1:4. ITG can be classified as either primary or secondary. Primary ITG (<1%) arises from aberrant thyroid tissue ectopically located in the mediastinum, receiving blood supply from mediastinal vessels and not connected to the cervical thyroid. Secondary ITG develops from the thyroid located in its normal cervical site; negative intra-thoracic pressure, gravity, and traction forces during swallowing facilitate downward migration of the thyroid into the mediastinum. The most common symptoms (dyspnea, choking, inability to sleep comfortably, dysphagia, and hoarseness) are related to compression of the airways and the esophagus. Less commonly, signs of compression of vascular and nervous structures are present, such as superior vena cava obstruction and/or Horner's syndrome. The diagnosis of ITG is based upon clinical history and examinations, and imaging findings. Nowadays CT scanning is the most comprehensive examination for the assessment of ITG extension and compression effects on adjacent anatomical structures. Surgical operations on large ITG are a major challenge in endocrine surgery. Surgery for ITG is required for the management of compression symptoms, potential airway compromise, and for the treatment of thyroid malignancy. While most ITG can be resected through a cervical approach, additional incisions, as manubriotomy, sternotomy, and lateral or antero-lateral thoracotomy, may be required. Lateral thoracotomy gives excellent exposure for a large posterior mediastinal goiter placed posterior to trachea with a crossover from the left side to the right side. During ITG operation, furthermore, there is a relevant rate of complications. The most frequent complication is the recurrent laryngeal nerve injury; the visual recognition of recurrent laryngeal nerve and a precise operative technique are still the most important factors for a successful operation. Another complication is parathyroid injury or blood supply impairment leading to postoperative hypocalcaemia. Postoperative hemorrhage is a rare but potentially fatal complication, occurring in 0.3 – 2%. In conclusion, in the presence of an ITG, extra-cervical access approach should be considered. The assessment and surgical treatment of ITG should be performed in specialized centers.

Chapter 3 – Hyperthyroidism is a common condition. Its prevalence is around 2% of women and 0.2% of men. Graves' disease is the most common cause of hyperthyroidism. There are three main approaches to treat hyperthyroidism: antithyroid drugs (ATD), radioiodine and surgery. Surgery and radioactive iodine are two types of ablative treatments. The selection of the suitable treatment depends on a number of factors such as etiology of the dysfunction, patient's age, associated comorbidities, and potential complications. Overall in Europe, ATD are usually offered whereas in the USA the first option is normally the radioiodine therapy. Regardless of the surgical technique, any patient who is undergoing surgery should be pretreated with ATD until the patient is in euthyroid state. Thyroidectomy has suffered major changes in terms of technique and incidence of complications in the past years. Many studies in the literature correlate the complications of thyroid surgery with the surgeon's experience.

Surgical procedures: Total thyroidectomy is the recommended procedure for definitive treatment in Graves' disease, and does not increase the rate of complications compared to lobectomy in the hands of experienced surgeons. In addition, total thyroidectomy minimizes the risk of relapse. Currently there are minimally invasive techniques such as endoscopic and video-assisted thyroidectomy. These techniques have been adopted by several centers, especially in Asia and Europe. The indications include benign thyroid disease and hyperthyroidism with a relatively small thyroid volume. Endoscopic robotic thyroidectomy by axillary approach is a new technique that has some cosmetic advantages. This technique offers an excellent operative field, allowing the identification of the vital structures.

Indications: Several situations such as pregnancy, reactions to ATD, rejection of radioiodine treatment, presence of Graves' ophthalmopathy, relapsed, and large goiter are some of the appropriate circumstances for surgery approach in hyperthyroidism.

Potential Complications: Thyroidectomy is associated with several complications such as: hypoparathyroidism (3.7% [0,6-50%]), recurrent laryngeal nerve damage (1-8%) which can be transient (2.5-3% [0,9-4,7%]) or permanent (0.3-2% [0-1,7%]), local hemorrhage (0.36%) which can cause laryngeal edema (4.3%, [1-1,3%]), thyrotoxic storm (1-2%), surgical site infection (0,5-3%) and recurrent hyperthyroidism (2%).

Conclusion: Although effective treatments for hyperthyroidism are available, none is perfect. Thyroid surgery is associated to negligible mortality and low complication rate. The experience of the surgeon and the use of new, less invasive techniques, reduce the risk of postoperative complications and improve the rate of recurrence.

Chapter 4 – Thyroidectomy is a well standardized procedure. Currently mortality rate is reduced close to zero and its complications are not worrisome. Technical progress and wide attention to the cosmetic results have pushed the development of new surgical techniques, namely Minimal Invasive Video Assisted thyroidectomy (MIVAT) and transaxillary robotic thyroidectomy. MIVAT can be considered a miniaturization of traditional cervicotomic approach with a similar spectrum of complications. In the literature have been described a subcutaneous reimplant from a benign goiter. With the transaxillary approach the spectrum of complications have been broadened with tunnel associated problems and the position of the arm. One of the authors (MP) have observed a neoplastic reimplant in the tunnel. The main complications of the classic thyroidectomy are:

- Acute post-operative hemorrage with compressive hematoma: this causes asphyxia, that requests emergency decompression. When bleeding is less dramatic we observe a subcutaneous hematoma, which determines a visible lump without respiratory problems
- Hypocalcemia is routinely checked and can be symptomatic or a laboratory diagnosis, associated with overt symptoms or not. The asymptomatic one can be a mild form of hypoparathyroidism, deserving some forms of treatment or can reflect a low protein level: this does not deserve any treatment.
- Recurrent laryngeal nerve injury can be transient or permanent, unilateral or bilateral: the last is one of the most dramatic acute event

in thyroid surgery. In the recent years many surgeons have suggested the use of neuromonitoring (NIM) to reduce the incidence of nerve palsy and more to avoid bilateral palsy with a staged thyroidectomy.

Other complication of thyroid surgery are:

- wound problems, like seroma, infection, cutaneous sensitive neck problems and a bad scar
- swallowing disorders
- chilous fistula
- Horner syndrome
- tracheal or esophageal injury

Further peculiar complications are associated to the dissection of lateral compartment of the neck.

Chapter 5 – The first thyroidectomy was performed in Baghdad circa 500 BC, but it was not until Emile Theodor Kocher refined his operative technique in the nineteenth century that it became accepted as a mainstream operative procedure. Due to the intricate relationship of numerous important functional structures in the neck, thyroidectomy was still fraught with life altering, and sometimes life threatening, complications. Despite this, surgical intervention for thyroid disease remains as one of the pillars of treatment with 80,000 thyroidectomies being performed in the United States annually.

The authors reviewed the surgical anatomy of the thyroid gland along with its relations to the parathyroid glands, recurrent and external laryngeal nerves in a prior chapter in this book. Anatomic variations were discussed as well as tips and tricks to identify these important structures at the time of surgery.

The indications for thyroidectomy together with the necessary pre-operative assessment including history, examination, thyroid function tests, ultrasound and fine needle aspiration cytology will be reviewed. The role of Computerised Tomography scan, radionucleotide scanning and Magnetic Resonance Imaging will be mentioned.

Traditional thyroid surgery involved the use of cold steel. In this era, bleeding was a major concern as the vessels are numerous and thin walled and they may retract to make control difficult. With the introduction of monopolar and bipolar diathermy operative time has decreased. Operative time and blood loss are even shorter now with the use of ultrasonic dissectors. Other tools including nerve stimulators will be discussed and the data analysed.

Recent advances in surgical equipment has fostered an evolution of the traditional thyroidectomy technique using sub-platysmal flaps. Considering that cosmesis remains one of the main indications for this operation, the authors have witnessed the introduction of video assisted thyroidectomy and robotic thyroidectomy. These minimally invasive techniques are explored, including their cost-benefit ratios and learning curves.

The authors also discuss modifications of the traditional open technique including the retrograde sub-capsular approach that facilitates preservation of the external branch of the superior laryngeal nerve when removing large bulky glands. They also strive to discuss means to prevent complications, treat them and look at the long term outcomes.

Chapter 6 – The first reports of thyroid surgery can be traced back to the 12th century, when only crude operative methods and rudimentary anaesthetic techniques were available. Theodor Kocher revolutionized the thyroiddectomy technique in 1877 by introducing meticulous dissection and better antisepsis techniques.

In the 1890's William Halsted, Charles Mayo and George Crile popularized Kocher's techniques in the United States.

Operative morbidity reduced further with technical refinements made by Thomas Dunhill who introduced capsular dissection in 1912 and Frank Lahey who popularized nerve preservation in 1938.

By the late 20th century there were significant advances in pharmacology, anaesthetic techniques and antisepsis. Coupled with refined operative techniques and meticulous dissection, thyroidectomy is now a safe operation with complication rates less than 1%.

To ensure good outcomes, surgeons performing thyroidectomy must be acutely familiar with the anatomy, and common variations of the thyroid gland. In this chapter the authors review the gross anatomy of the gland, with special emphasis on the surgical importance of the structures encountered during a thyroidectomy. The authors discuss the anatomic basis of the operative techniques and the common variations that may be encountered when performing a thyroidectomy.

Chapter 7 – Thyroid surgery is traditionally performed using Kocher incision over the neck for years. With the development of minimal access surgical equipment, there are a variety of surgical methods to achieve thyroid surgery with a good cosmetic result. These include cervical approach by means of minimally invasive video-assisted thyroidectomy using a mini-incision in the neck, or extra-cervical approach by means of remote access via the breast, chest wall and/or axilla. With the use of da Vinci Robotic Surgical

System, the authors would expect this operation to be performed under a steady, magnified and high definition videoscopic view at a higher surgical cost.

In this chapter, the author will discuss various methods of endoscopic thyroidectomy. Indication, surgical procedure and potential benefits of each procedure will be highlighted. They will also share their own series of endoscopic and robotic thyroidectomy. The potential complications and special precautions will be discussed as well. The authors hope their reader will have an overview on endoscopic and robotic thyroidectomy after reading this chapter.

Chapter 8 – A review of 814 thyroid surgery performed in a Public Hospital at Buenos Aires is presented in order to compare the authors' statistic with international reports. They compare sex, age, pathology, histological type, surgical procedures, complications and associated treatment to surgery in malignant tumors.

In: Thyroidectomy
Editor: Kimberly Rodolfo

ISBN: 978-1-63321-440-8

Chapter 1

The Clinical Utility of Serum Thyrotrophin Receptor Antibodies (TRAb) – An Update for Surgeons

***L. N. R. Bondugulapati*[1], *M. A. Adlan*[2] *and L. D. Premawardhana*[1,2*]**

[1]Centre for Endocrine and Diabetes Sciences,
University Hospital of Wales, Heath Park, Cardiff;
[2]Section of Endocrinology, Department of Medicine,
Ysbyty Ystrad Fawr, Ystrad Fawr Way, Hengoed, UK

Abstract

The immunopathogenesis of Graves' disease (GD) is an evolving story, but the central role of Thyrotrophin receptor antibodies (TRAb) in its aetiology is well established. TRAb are primarily produced in intrathyroidal immune competent cells. In treatment naïve subjects, they are found as stimulating (TSAb), blocking (TBAb) or possible neutral TRAb. The clinical phenotype is therefore dependent on the dominant form in the blood i.e. GD when TSAb, and hypothyroidism when TBAb predominates. But currently

* Corresponding author: Dr. L.D. Premawardhana. Email – premawardhanald@cardiff.ac.uk.

commercially available assays in clinical use cannot differentiate between TSAb and TBAb and there is no consensus about the utility of TRAb, in diagnosing or predicting outcome in GD.

There are two assay types used to measure TRAb – "receptor assays" and "bioassays". Although these assays can detect TRAb in up to 95% of GD patients, only the currently relatively cumbersome, time consuming and more expensive bioassay can determine their functional characteristics. Their clinical utility is therefore limited to research. The more user friendly, easy to perform and cheaper receptor assays measure both TSAb and TBAb, and cannot differentiate between them. Therefore TRAb positivity in these assays does not predict clinical phenotype or outcome. Complicating these analytical imperfections, TRAb also has the ability to change from one type to the other during the course of the disease and its treatment. The clinician therefore has only an imperfect tool to diagnose and predict GD outcome.

TRAb measurement in clinical situations other than isolated GD, merits discussion - (a) GD complicates pregnancy in a minority and the utility of maternal TRAb measurement to predict foetal and neonatal problems due to tranpslacental TRAb transfer is well established. (b) The recently described "Immune reconstitution syndrome" in patients receiving drugs such as Alemtuzumab and the highly active anti retrovirals (HAART), predisposes affected individuals to GD, and TRAb assays help diagnosis. (c) The occurrence of typical Graves' orbitopathy (GO) in hypothyroid and euthyroid patients and (d) unilateral GO are also situations where TRAb measurement helps.

Introduction

Graves' disease (GD) is one of the commonest causes of hyperthyroidism in the West. GD primarily affects the thyroid, and in some, the eyes and skin. But secondary involvement of the heart, bones, and other organs is well known and contributes to its morbidity [1]. It is characterised by the presence of autoantibodies against the Thyrotrophin receptor (TSHR), detectable in up to 95 % of affected individuals using current assays [2]. These Thyrotrophin receptor antibodies (TRAb) are produced in intrathyroidal immune competent cells. Their role in the pathogenesis of GD is well defined and is related to their ability to bind the TSH receptor, and stimulate it in a manner analogous to TSH. Measurement of TRAb in subjects suspected of having GD should therefore assist in its diagnosis, as it is so closely involved in its pathogenesis.

However, the link between detectable TRAb in the serum, and the clinical manifestations of GD and its outcome, is an unpredictable one. This relates to the variable ability of naturally occurring TRAb to stimulate the TSHR, as much as to the imperfections of current assay methodology. It is known that TRAb can be of different "functional" types based on their ability to activate the TSHR – stimulating, blocking and the recently described "neutral" antibody types [3]. A predominance of stimulating TRAb (TSAb) in the blood results in GD; and a predominance of blocking TRAb (TBAb), results in hypothyroidism. The balance between their opposing actions, therefore determines the clinical phenotype at presentation. Confusingly for the practising clinician, commonly available commercial TRAb assays do not differentiate between these "functional" types of TRAb, and cannot predict the clinical phenotype or the outcome of GD. There is no consensus therefore about the clinical utility of TRAb assays in diagnosing and managing GD.

We discuss in this chapter, TRAb assay methodology and their relevance to clinical practice, the natural history of TRAb during and after treatment of GD, and the clinical utility of measuring TRAb in diagnosing and predicting the outcome of GD.

TRAb Assay Methodology

There are two currently available assay methods for measuring serum TRAb in the clinical and research settings –

Receptor assays – these are freely available commercially, and are the assays used in clinical practice [4]. These assays detect TRAb by their ability to compete with a TSH receptor (TSHR) ligand (e.g. radiolabelled TSH or anti-TSHR monoclonal antibodies) for binding sites on the TSHR. They therefore detect "thyroid binding inhibiting immunoglobulins" (TBII), without clarifying their "functional properties", i.e. they do not differentiate between TSAb and TBAb. Consequently, their existence in the serum does not predict accurately either the clinical phenotype or the outcome of GD as TRAb positive individuals may have a combination of TSAb and TBAb and at any given time the predominant form would determine the clinical phenotype.

Receptor assays have undergone considerable modification and development over the decades. The early, imprecise, first generation porcine and bovine assays using liquid phase technology, were largely superseded by second generation, solid phase, recombinant human TSHR based assays. They used ELISA techniques and chemiluminescence instead of radioactive readouts as their end points. They were highly sensitive and specific in some studies. However, third generation assays using human monoclonal TSHR stimulating antibodies are even better according to some recent evidence. TRAb assays are fully automated and are suited well for clinical use.

Bioassays – these assays use cultured cells, and measure cAMP production as an indicator of TSHR stimulation by TRAb in the serum. They are mostly used in the research setting. While first generation bioassays used human, porcine and rat thyroid cell lines (with intact TSHR), second-generation tests made use of Chinese hamster ovary cells transfected with human TSHR. Third generation bioassays use a luciferase reporter gene to generate light in more simplified assays. Further modifications to these have utilised chimeric human TSHR and rat luteinizing hormone (LH) receptors (the rat LH elements replacing TBAb binding epitopes in the wild type TSHR). These changes are thought to have increased assay sensitivity and simplified it from a practical point of view [5]. These bioassays have the ability to differentiate between TSAb and TBAb, but are currently not commonly used in daily clinical practice.

We have highlighted the features of receptor and bioassays and their clinical use in Table 1.

Table 1. Features of the two types of TRAb assays currently available

Receptor Assays	Bioassays
Easily available for clinical use	Mostly a research tool at present
Cheaper and easy to do, with high sensitivity	More time consuming, cumbersome, labour intensive and currently more expensive
Don’t differentiate between TSAb and TBAb	Differentiate between TSAb and TBAb
May lack correlation with clinical phenotype and severity of illness	
Limited use in predicting outcome	

TRAb Concentration and Treatment of GD

All three current treatment modalities for GD – thionamides (methimazole, carbimazole, propylthiouracil), radioactive iodine (RAI) and surgery - reduce TRAb concentration in the serum. The time course of this decrease and its extent are variable [6]. The reason for this decrease in TRAb when GD is treated is unclear, but treatment induced immune modulation (particularly with thionamide therapy and surgery) and controlling biochemical hyperthyroidism (by all three modalities) are the main contenders. The immune modulatory effects of thionamide therapy are well described. Surgery too results in some immune modulation by antigen (TSHR) removal and by inducing T and B lymphocyte apoptosis by sudden intense antigen release during surgery. The predictable smooth TRAb reduction that should therefore occur with these two treatment modalities is actually borne out in clinical practice [6]. RAI induces a different pattern of change to serum TRAb levels. An initial sudden increase in TRAb, most likely due to RAI induced tissue destruction and antigen release, is followed by a slower and more incomplete reduction of TRAb over many years. RAI also has effects on T regulatory cells, which contribute to its mild immune modulatory properties. The change to TRAb concentrations during treatment described above would suggest that the persistence of high levels of TRAb after treatment would predict a recurrence of GD. But the story is far from clear.

The Clinical Utility of TRAb Assays in Diagnosis and Prediction of Outcome

- TRAb in the differential diagnosis of thyrotoxicosis

Graves' disease - The major clinical use for TRAb measurement in clinical practice is in confirming the diagnosis of GD. However, despite a very simple and clear relationship between TRAb and the clinical manifestations of GD, its use as a diagnostic tool remains variable. This is partly because professional societies have been slow in responding to the evidence [7], and also because of differing practice across the world. The American Thyroid Association (ATA) and the American Association of Clinical Endocrinologists (AACE) both recommend RAI uptake scans as first line investigation for thyrotoxicosis [8]. The British Thyroid Association (BTA) in their 2006 guidelines recommended TRAb testing only in special situations [9]. This is surprising as TRAb testing where it is established as a first line test (most European centres), is "user friendly" for the patient (a single blood test at the time of clinic visit), has a much quicker turnaround time (a few days compared to several weeks for RAI uptake scans) and is considerably cheaper. Furthermore, third generation receptor assays are very sensitive and specific with high positive and negative predictive values and therefore clinicians can use them with confidence. It is our practice to use TRAb assays as a first line test in the differential diagnosis of thyrotoxicosis.

Toxic Nodular Disease

Subjects with toxic nodular disease are almost all TRAb negative. In appropriate circumstances (clinically thyrotoxic patients with nodular goitres) a negative TRAb test would indicate the need for further investigations (e.g. a RAI uptake scan) and facilitate definitive treatment at an early stage.

"Thyroiditis"

Several conditions causing a "destructive thyroiditis" give rise to mild and short lasting thyrotoxicosis, which is usually self-limiting. Subacute or De Quervain's thyroiditis, painless thyroiditis, postpartum thyroiditis (PPT) and some forms of drug-induced thyroiditis fall in to this category. Their mild clinical presentation, combined with the absence of serum TRAb, help in eliminating GD as a cause. Furthermore, RAI uptake is low or absent in these subjects. The use of colour flow Doppler analysis also may help to differentiate these conditions from the more "vascular" looking thyroid gland found in GD. RAI uptake or colour flow Doppler scans would help in the small percentage of patients with some forms of destructive thyroiditis who are also TRAb positive.

The "Immune Reconstitution Syndrome" –

Modern treatment of multiple sclerosis (MS) and HIV disease, using drugs that cause lymphocyte depletion (Alemtuzumab, an anti-CD52 monoclonal antibody in MS; and highly active antiretroviral therapy or HAART in HIV infection), causes the recently described "Immune reconstitution syndrome" in a significant minority of individuals, estimated to be about 30% in MS (10). This syndrome may occur in bone marrow transplantation too. Antigen naïve CD4 cell expansion during the phase of "reconstitution" following initial lymphocyte depletion, results in TRAb formation, when these "antigen naïve" immune competent cells are exposed to thyroid antigens, and results in GD in these subjects.

- TRAb in the prediction of GD outcome

A clinical tool that could predict the natural history of GD at an early stage in its clinical course e.g. at first clinical presentation, would be of benefit to both patients and clinicians. Knowledge of the clinical course of GD in each patient (e.g. would there be remission or recurrence after stopping anti thyroid drugs) may help avoid prolonged treatment with potentially complicated medication regimes with significant side effects. Definitive treatment with RAI or surgery could then be recommended for those likely to have a recurrence, at an early stage of their illness.

An ideal prediction tool should be easy and cheap to measure, sensitive, and have high positive and negative predictive values when measured in the initial stages of the disease. Early attempts at predicting the course of the disease used clinical data (goitre volume, family history of GD, age, gender, smoking etc.), biochemical data (thyroid hormone levels) or immunological data (TRAb levels, rate of TRAb decline during treatment, etc.) either singly or in combination, but were not entirely satisfactory. Most subsequent studies have used TRAb as the prediction tool of choice in view of its intimate link to the pathogenesis of GD. We have summarised the studies examining TRAb in this role published within the last decade or so in Table 2. Although there were a handful of studies where persistent and elevated TRAb concentrations were predictive of early relapse (6 months and 56 weeks respectively in two studies), its utility in predicting GD remission/relapse is still unproven. The lack of large, reproducible, well-designed, prospective studies is a shortcoming in this area of thyroidology. The variable study design, TRAb assay methodology used, and target study populations in studies depicted, and the variability of the intrinsic molecular and functional characteristics of the TRAb molecule (both TSAb and TBAb found in the serum of most TRAb positive patients), and its ability to change from one form to the other, make this aspect of GD management frustrating and lacking in consensus. The jury is still out on the use of TRAb measurement as a predictive tool of GD recurrence [4, 7].

- TRAb measurement in special situations

(1) Pregnancy

The majority of subjects who develop hyperthyroidism during pregnancy have GD – estimated to be about 85% in total. The immune modulation that occurs in the mother to accommodate the foetus (which is a “foreign body” with paternal antigens), has a salutary effect on GD too. TRAb levels fall and the disease becomes easier to control, and in some completely remits in the third trimester. In some however, TRAb levels continue to be high in late pregnancy.

Table 2. Recent clinical studies examining the utility of TRAb assays in predicting GD outcome

Author [year, (ref)]	Assay (n)	Study design	TRAb cut Off value	% Relapse	PPV %
Zimmerman-Belsing [2002, [12]]	TBII (129)	TRAb assays at diagnosis (122) and at withdrawal of drugs (129) – median follow up 18 months	1.5 U/l	45	49
Quadbeck [2005, [13]]	TBII (96)	TRAb assays done 4 weeks after withdrawal of drugs – follow up for 2 years in total	1.5 U/l 10 U/l	49	49 83
Quadbeck [2005, [13]]	Bioassay (96)	As above	1.5 U/l		49 TSAb - 51
Schott [2007, [14]]	TBII (131)	TRAb and TPOAb assays done 4.3 months (mean) after GD diagnosis	>2 and <6 U/l >6+>5000 >6+ >500	71.8	66.7-90 100 93.7-96
Capelli [2007, [15]]	TBII (216)	TRAb assays done at diagnosis and 6 monthly for 10 years	>46.5 U/l at diagnosis or >30.7 U/l at 6 months	67.1	52% 53.2%
Massart [2009, [16])	TBII (128)	TRAb assays compared after 18 months of treatment - 3 year follow up	0.94 – 3.2 IU/l	48	53-66%
Giuliani (2012, [17])	Bioassay Mc4 chimera (55)	TSAb at diagnosis in those who had remission, relapse and unsuspended therapy – 5 year follow up		49 (relapse and unsuspended therapy)	95.4%

These TRAb can travel transplacentally and cause intrauterine problems for the foetus by stimulating its thyroid gland – foetal tachycardia, growth retardation etc. TRAb is a predictor of such foetal and neonatal problems and its measurement helps in managing children of mothers with GD, both during the intrauterine and neonatal phases. Pregnant mothers on anti thyroid medication, those who have had RAI or surgery previously for GD, and those who have given birth to children with neonatal thyrotoxicosis should have serum TRAb checked. TRAb should definitely be checked in the third trimester, but some would limit this to those who were positive in the first trimester [11].

(2) Euthyroid, Hypothyroid or Unilateral GO

Although sight-threatening GO occurs in only about 5% of subjects with GD, a significant proportion will have clinical evidence of eye involvement – estimated to be between 30-50% in some studies. When clinical symptoms and signs of GD co-exist with signs of GO, it is easy to make an accurate diagnosis. However, serum TRAb needs to be measured when GO occurs (a) without clinical symptoms or signs of GD – euthyroid GO, (b) in hypothyroid patients – hypothyroid GO, and (c) in one eye only – unilateral GO.

Table 3. Current indications for TRAb testing

Indications for TRAb testing
(1) Establishing diagnosis of GD and differentiating from other thyrotoxic conditions
(2) Euthyroid or hypothyroid orbitopathy
(3) Unilateral orbitopathy
(4) Pregnancy in women who –
(a) are currently on anti thyroid drug therapy
(b) have had ablative therapy for GD (RAI or surgery)
(c) have given birth to children with neonatal thyrotoxicosis
TRAb to be checked in the first trimester and at 22-26 weeks gestation
(5) Thyrotoxicosis complicating the Immune reconstitution syndrome (use of CAMPATH and HAART)

Conclusion

Assay imperfections, and the intrinsic variability of the functional properties of the TRAb molecule (e.g. found in two forms in the serum –

TSAb and TBAb), make it an imperfect tool both for the diagnosis and for the prediction of outcome of GD. Such a tool would be very useful for clinicians managing patients with GD, to tailor treatment to the individual patient. Despite these imperfections, TRAb remains a clinically useful investigative tool in the differential diagnosis of the thyrotoxic state. In the appropriate clinical setting, TRAb positivity establishes the diagnosis of GD in up to 95% of patients. However, its utility in predicting the outcome of GD remains unresolved and there is no consensus currently.

TRAb measurements using current 3rd generation "receptor" assays are freely available, easily and relatively quickly done, and indeed cheap to do in high volume laboratories. They offer a higher degree of sensitivity and specificity over thyroid peroxidase antibodies (another thyroid antibody recommended by some experts), a quicker turnaround time compared to RAI uptake scans (recommended by some specialist societies) and are definitely cheaper. We have summarised in Table 3 the current indications for TRAb testing in clinical practice.

In conclusion we feel that although the value of TRAb measurement using current assays, in predicting the outcome of GD remains unresolved, we believe its use in diagnosing GD and differentiating between the causes of thyrotoxicosis is firmly established.

References

[1] F. Menconi, C. Marcocci, M. Marinò. Diagnosis and classification of Graves' disease. *Autoimmun. Rev.* 2014; 14: 398-402.

[2] K. Zophel, D. Roggenbuck, M. Schott, Clinical review about TRAb assay's history. *Autoimmun. Rev.* 2010; 9: 695–700.

[3] S. A. Morshed, T. Ando, R. Latif, T. F. Davies, Neutral antibodies to the TSH receptor are present in Graves' disease and regulate selective signaling cascades. *Endocrinol.* 2010; 151: 5537–5549.

[4] C. Kamath, M. A. Adlan, L. D. Premawardhana. The role of Thyrotorophin receptor antibody assays in Graves' disease. *J. Thy. Res.* 2012; 525936: 1-8.

[5] S.D. Lytton, G.J. Kahaly. Bioassays for TSH-receptor autoantibodies: an update. *Autoimmun. Rev.* 2010; 10: 116–122.

[6] P. Laurberg, G. Wallin, L. Tallstedt, M. Abraham-Nordling, G. Lundell, O. Tørring. TSH -receptor autoimmunity in Graves' disease after therapy

with anti-thyroid drugs, surgery, or radioiodine: a 5-year prospective randomized study. *Eur. J. Endocrinol.* 2008; 158: 69-75.

[7] G. Barbesino, Y. Tomer. Clinical Utility of TSH Receptor Antibodies. *J. Clin. Endocrinol. Metab.* 2013; 98: 2247–2255.

[8] R. S. Bahn, H. B. Burch, D. S. Cooper, et al. Hyperthyroidism and other causes of thyrotoxicosis: management guidelines of the American Thyroid Association and American Association of Clinical Endocrinologists. *Thyroid* 2011; 21: 593–646.

[9] G. H. Beastall, G. J. Beckett, J. A. Franklyn et al; British Thyroid Association. UK Guidelines for the use of thyroid function tests. http://www.british thyroid association.org/info for patients/Docs/ TFT_guideline_final_version_July_2006.pdf. Accessed May 2013.

[10] P. Weetman. Graves' disease following immune reconstitution or immunomodulatory treatment: should we manage it any differently. *Clin. Endocrinol. (Oxf)* 2014; 80: 629-32.

[11] J. H. Lazarus, L. D. Premawardhana. Thyroid disease during pregnancy. Oxford Textbook of Endocrinology (Oxford University Press, Oxford). Eds. J. A. H. Wass, P. M. Stewart, S. Amiel, M. Davies. 2011; chapter 345: 527-532.

[12] T. Zimmermann-Belsing, B. Nygaard, A. K. Rasmussen, U. Feldt-Rasmussen. Use of the 2nd generation TRAK human assay did not improve prediction of relapse after antithyroid medical therapy of Graves' disease. *Eur. J. Endocrinol.* 2002; 146: 173–177.

[13] B. Quadbeck, R. Hoermann, U. Roggenbuck, S. Hahn, K. Mann, and O. E. Janssen. Sensitive thyrotrophin and thyrotrophin-receptor antibody determinations one month after discontinuation of antithyroid drug treatment as predictors of relapse in Graves' disease. *Thyroid.* 2005; 15: 1047– 1054.

[14] M.Schott, A.Eckstein, H.S.Willenberg, T.B.T.Nguyen, N.G. Morgenthaler, W. A. Scherbaum. Improved prediction of relapse of Graves' thyrotoxicosis by combined determination of TSH receptor and thyroperoxidase antibodies. *Horm. Metab. Res.* 2007; 39: 56–61.

[15] C. Cappelli, E. Gandossi, M. Castellano et al., Prognostic value of thyrotropin receptor antibodies (TRAb) in Graves' disease: a 120 months prospective study. *Endocr. J.* 2007; 54: 713–720.

[16] C.Massart, J.Gibassier, M.d'Herbomen. Clinical value of M22-based assays for TSH-receptor antibody (TRAb) in the follow-up of antithyroid drug treated Graves' disease: comparison with the second generation human TRAb assay *Clin. Chim. Acta.* 2009; 407: 62–6.

[17] C. Giuliani, D. Cerrone, N. Harii, M. Thornton, L.D. Kohn, N.M. Dagia, E. Fiore, I. Bucci, T. Chamblin, P. Vitti, F. Monaco, G. Napolitano. A TSHr-LH/CGr chimera that measures functional TSAb in Graves' disease. *J. Clin. Endocrinol. Metab.* 2012; 97: E1106-15.

In: Thyroidectomy
Editor: Kimberly Rodolfo

ISBN: 978-1-63321-440-8

Chapter 2

Thyroidectomy for Intrathoracic Goiter: Surgical Procedures, Potential Complications and Postoperative Outcomes

Luca Bertolaccini*[*1], Andrea Viti[1], Corrado Lauro[2] and Alberto Terzi[3]
[1]Thoracic Surgery Unit, S. Croce e Carle Hospital, Cuneo, Italy
[2]Section of Endocrine Surgery, S. Croce e Carle Hospital, Cuneo, Italy
[3]Section of Thoracic Surgery, Sacred Heart Hospital, Negrar, Verona, Italy

Abstract

Albrecht von Haller first described an Intra-Thoracic Goiter (ITG) in 1749. Terms such as retrosternal, sub-sternal, intrathoracic, or mediastinal have also been used to define a goiter that extends beyond the thoracic inlet. Incidence in the general population, based on mass chest Computed Tomography (CT) screening, is 0.02 – 0.5%. The diagnosis of ITG is frequently made in the fifth or sixth decade of life, with a male/female

* Corresponding Author: Luca Bertolaccini, MD PhD FCCP. Mailing address: Thoracic Surgery Unit, S. Croce e Carle Hospital, Via Michele Coppino 26 – 12100 Cuneo (IT). Tel:+39-0171-641450; Fax: +39-0171-642491; E-Mail: luca.bertolaccini@gmail.com.

rate of 1:4. ITG can be classified as either primary or secondary. Primary ITG (<1%) arises from aberrant thyroid tissue ectopically located in the mediastinum, receiving blood supply from mediastinal vessels and not connected to the cervical thyroid. Secondary ITG develops from the thyroid located in its normal cervical site; negative intra-thoracic pressure, gravity, and traction forces during swallowing facilitate downward migration of the thyroid into the mediastinum. The most common symptoms (dyspnea, choking, inability to sleep comfortably, dysphagia, and hoarseness) are related to compression of the airways and the esophagus. Less commonly, signs of compression of vascular and nervous structures are present, such as superior vena cava obstruction and/or Horner's syndrome. The diagnosis of ITG is based upon clinical history and examinations, and imaging findings. Nowadays CT scanning is the most comprehensive examination for the assessment of ITG extension and compression effects on adjacent anatomical structures. Surgical operations on large ITG are a major challenge in endocrine surgery. Surgery for ITG is required for the management of compression symptoms, potential airway compromise, and for the treatment of thyroid malignancy. While most ITG can be resected through a cervical approach, additional incisions, as manubriotomy, sternotomy, and lateral or antero-lateral thoracotomy, may be required. Lateral thoracotomy gives excellent exposure for a large posterior mediastinal goiter placed posterior to trachea with a crossover from the left side to the right side. During ITG operation, furthermore, there is a relevant rate of complications. The most frequent complication is the recurrent laryngeal nerve injury; the visual recognition of recurrent laryngeal nerve and a precise operative technique are still the most important factors for a successful operation. Another complication is parathyroid injury or blood supply impairment leading to postoperative hypocalcaemia. Postoperative hemorrhage is a rare but potentially fatal complication, occurring in 0.3 – 2%. In conclusion, in the presence of an ITG, extra-cervical access approach should be considered. The assessment and surgical treatment of ITG should be performed in specialized centers.

Introduction

In 1749, Albrecht von Haller described in his paper the Intra-Thoracic Goiter (ITG), as extension of thyroidal tissue below the suprasternal notch (*fossa jugularis sternalis*) [1]. Since there are technical hitches that may be encountered during surgical removal, ITG is a challenge for general surgeons. A widely accepted definition of ITG is still lacking. Usually ITG refers to a goiter that is for at least 50% located in the mediastinum [2 – 3]. Other definitions of ITG have been suggested:

1. A thyroid in which any part of the gland extends below the thoracic inlet with the patient in the surgical position [4];
2. A gland reaching the level of the aortic arch [5];
3. A thyroid reaching the level of T4 (on chest roentgenogram) [6];
4. Greater than 50% of the gland residing below the thoracic inlet [2].

Although there are arguments for and against the use of each definition, surgeons should develop a common definition to compare patients and results.

Epidemiology and Classification

The incidence of ITG is variable (from 2 to 19% of all thyroidectomies) [7 – 9]. The clinical diagnosis is most frequently made in the fifth or sixth decade of life (ratio female/male = 4:1). The ITG can be primary or secondary.

Primary ITG is very rare (1%), it arises from thyroid tissue ectopically located in the mediastinum due to an abnormal embryologic migration anlage closely associated with the aortic sac; it receives the blood supply from mediastinal vessels and it has no connection with the thyroid.

Secondary ITG develops from the normal cervical thyroid; the migration into the mediastinum is facilitated by negative intra-thoracic pressure, gravity, swallowing traction forces and anatomical barriers that prevent the enlargement in other directions. The secondary ITG is in continuity with the cervical portion of thyroid and it receives the blood supply usually through branches of the inferior thyroid artery. Sometimes, ITG may extend cranially behind or along the side of the pharynx, but they may exceptionally extend even to the diaphragm [10 – 11]. Additional factors associated with ITG are short neck, short cervical trachea, and well-developed neck muscles [12].

Symptoms and Diagnosis

Usually patients with ITG complaint of a slow-growing but asymptomatic enlargement of the neck for many years; in about 30% of cases ITG are incidentally discovered with chest radiography [13]. The most common symptoms, related to compression of the upper aero-digestive ways, are represented by dyspnea, choking, inability to sleep comfortably, dysphagia and hoarseness. Less common signs are the superior vena cava syndrome and/or Horner's syndrome, both indirect evidences of the compression of vascular and nervous structures.

The diagnosis of ITG is based on history, clinical examinations, and imaging findings [14]. Computed Tomography (CT) scan of the neck and the chest is the gold standard for the assessment of extension of the goiter and the mass effect on adjacent structures [15].

Surgical Treatment

The presence of ITG is an indication for surgery in an otherwise healthy patient, even in the absence of clinical symptoms [16] because there is no effective treatment other than surgery, and because thyrodectomy, the treatment of choice, performed by skilled surgeons is both safe and effective. Alternative treatments such as thyroid hormone ablation or radioactive iodine ablation are rarely successful [17 – 18]. Moreover, ITG can become a life-threatening emergency, if a sudden enlargement of goiter due to hemorrhage occurs. Furthermore, in 3 – 21% of ITG [19] thyroid cancer was detected into the goiter. Tracheomalacia on the contrary is an extremely rare complication as well as the superior vena cava syndrome and it is virtually nonexistent in thyroid glands extending just below the thoracic inlet. It is essential to identify preoperatively patients who could require a thoracic approach, in order to plan the presence of a multidisciplinary team with the thoracic surgeon, and to inform correctly the patient. As reported in Literature the thoracic approach is probable in ITG that are >70% in the mediastinum, in ITG >10 cm, in patients with a history of cervical thyroidectomy, and in patients with an invasive carcinoma or ectopic goiter [26]. Recently, four factors were identified that significantly increase the need of a thoracic approach for an ITG:

1. The presence of malignancy;
2. The involvement of the posterior mediastinum;
3. The extension of the ITG below the aortic arch;
4. The presence of ectopic goiter [22].

The removal of ITG is associated with higher morbidity and even mortality, especially when an extracervical thoracic approach is required [23].

To avoid a thoracotomy or a sternotomy, many techniques have been described to facilitate extraction. Accurate surgical technique that includes adequate cervical incision, proper strap muscles preparation, thyroid section, progressive traction over the upper pole to allow a safe delivery of the goiters extending into the mediastinum through a cervical approach [12]. Although the necessity of extracervical extension should be planned preoperatively, the decision to perform an extracervical access should always be made intraoperatively, after careful attempts to remove the mass through the cervical incision [24].

Surgical Technique

Total thyroidectomy is defined as total bilateral extracapsular thyroidectomy; hemithyroidectomy is defined as total unilateral extracapsular thyroidectomy; completion thyroidectomy is defined as the removal of all the residual thyroid tissue after previous unilateral or bilateral thyroid resections (nodulectomy, hemithyroidectomy, subtotal thyroidectomy) [22]. Most ITG can be removed through a proper cervical approach, while a thoracic approach should be performed only in few patients (1 – 11%) [25]; nevertheless some Authors have reported the need of a sternotomy in 29% [26]. This variability has to be correlated with the lack of uniformity in definition of ITG. After oral intubation, the patient is placed in a supine position with the neck well extended. Iodine-free solutions should be used to swab the operative fields. The Kocher's cervical transverse incision is performed 1 to 2 cm higher than usual to gain a better access to the gland. The strap muscles are usually divided along the midline. In selected cases, the strap muscles can be sectioned in order to obtain a better exposure and then they are reconstructed at the end of the operation. After mobilization of the upper pole, the superior thyroid vessels are ligated close to the thyroid capsule avoiding injury to the external branch of the superior laryngeal nerve, which is not routinely exposed. The middle thyroid vein is identified and ligated to allow the mobilization of the substernal extension. A systematic and prompt identification of the recurrent laryngeal nerves is mandatory in thyroid surgery, usually where they cross the inferior thyroid artery. After their identification, the surgeon should follow the recurrent laryngeal nerve upward until it enters the larynx. If the nerve is not found at its usual place, the surgeons should be aware of the possibility of a non-recurrent inferior laryngeal nerve on the right side. In some situation, the recurrent laryngeal nerve should be identified first at its entry point, which represents the most constant site, and then followed downward, before goiter delivery. The gland is then progressively delivered through the incision by gentle traction over the upper thyroid pole (the so called ''toboggan technique'') [25]. It has been suggested that digital luxation of the goiter be avoided because this maneuver poses recurrent nerves at risk in the case of nerves displacement by large goiters. In all the cases, an effort is made by the surgeons to identify and preserve all the parathyroid glands. Parathyroid auto-transplantation in the ipsilateral sternocleidomastoid muscle is performed only in the case of a compromised vascular supply or an inadvertent excision.

In patients with ITG, when cervicotomy is not adequate, the intrathoracic approaches that can be used are:

- Manubriotomy;
- Full sternotomy;
- Antero-lateral thoracotomy to the fourth intercostal space.

Manubriotomy, or full sternotomy, by vertical extension of the cervical incision can be performed rapidly and with very low morbidity, [27] and they provide excellent exposure of mediastinum to allow delivery of the retrosternal portion of the gland [28], and they can be performed without repositioning the patient [29]. A partial upper sternotomy is performed through a limited skin incision, extending less than 6 cm below the sternal notch. Gradual spreading of the sternal halves permits a complete exposure of the antero-superior mediastinum without sternal fracture and a self-retraining retractor is placed [26]. Extension to a total sternotomy can be performed when necessary.

Retrosternal extension of mediastinal goiters does not appear to be, per se, a predicting factor for sternal incision; while posterior mediastinum involvement by the gland is considered a strong predictor for the need of a thoracotomy [22]. ITG that descends into the posterior mediastinum behind the carotid sheath and recurrent laryngeal nerve can cause significant esophageal displacement and compression. These ITG are difficult to extract through a cervical approach alone, and even sternotomy affords suboptimal exposure. Therefore, posterior mediastinal extension can require thoracotomy in addition to the cervical incision [27].

Discussion

According to Hedayati [27], postoperative morbidity is more common after ITG resection than in standard thyrodectomy for cervical thyroid disease. Various risk factors for complications have been described, including longer operative time, increased blood loss, extension beyond the carina, or very large thyroid glands [28]. While the complications rate, both transient and definitive, was similar for patients operated on for ITG or cervical goiters according to others [12]. Conversely, operative time and mean hospital stay were longer in patients with ITG.

An accurate and appropriate surgical technique is mandatory. In particular, blind finger luxation of the thyroid lobe should be avoided in any case to reduce the risk of recurrent laryngeal nerve damage and dangerous and difficult-to-control mediastinal hemorrhages [29]. When dissection cannot be safely performed from a cervical incision, even after sectioning the strap muscles, an extracervical approach becomes mandatory. The need of an extracervical approach and the complication rates are highly correlated with the experience of the surgical team.

There is a consensus that the vast majority of ITG can be successfully removed through a cervical approach. Several series have examined the factors that increase the possibility of a thoracic approach. Thoracotomy or sternotomy is inevitable when a goiter is iceberg shaped and more than 70% of it resides within the mediastinum. According to literature a thoracic approach might be necessary for the malignant substernal goiter (although not mandatory), the posterior ITG with contralateral extension or mediastinal blood supply, the ITG causing superior vena cava syndrome, the reoperation cases, the occurrence of a significant mediastinal hemorrhage, and when the diameter of mediastinal goiter exceeds the thoracic inlet diameter [30]. The inlet has relatively fixed dimensions, as both the bony clavicle and sternum are unyielding. Pressure against the partially distensible trachea will permit temporary but only slight enlargement of the inlet [31]. Although malignancy does not automatically mandate sternotomy, thoracic access should be considered when adhesion to mediastinal structures or blood vessels is preoperatively detected or suspected and for larger cancers whose transit through the thoracic inlet might result in tumor spillage [32]. The most important predictive factor as to whether a goiter can safely be removed through a cervical approach is the presence of a clear tissue plane in the mediastinum on preoperative imaging [33].

The growth of a thyroid in the neck or chest can be considerable without causing severe tracheal compression, but growth in the inlet can wedge the goiter between the rigid manubrium and the cartilaginous trachea. Enlargement of the goiter in the inlet can therefore cause severe tracheal compression. Moreover, these patients often cannot extend their heads during intubation, since the maneuver will elevate the mediastinal part of the goiter into the inlet and result in tracheal narrowing. Thus while a large goiter located inferiorly in the mediastinum can sometimes be completely asymptomatic [34], a smaller goiter located at the thoracic inlet may cause severe symptoms.

Conclusion

Thyrodectomy for an ITG can be safely performed through a cervical incision in most patients. A thoracic approach has very limited indications and should be used in selected patients. Preoperative CT or MRI scans help to select these patients. Posterior mediastinal involvement, the massive size of a goiter extending inferior to the aortic arch, and an ectopic goiter located deep in the mediastinum are factors posed for the patients at risk of sternotomy or thoracotomy. An extracervical approach does not increase the morbidity of surgery and may be "safer surgery" in selected conditions. ITG should be operated on in high volume specialized centers to obtain the best results, as surgery, in this case, does not seem to be associated with a higher risk of postoperative complications.

References

[1] Haller A. *Disputatones Anatomica Selectae.* Gottingen:Vendenhoceck; 1749. p. 96.

[2] deSouza FM, Smith PE. Retrosternal goiter. *J Otolaryngol* 1983;12:393-396.

[3] Katlic MR, Wang CA, Grillo HC. Substernal goiter. *Ann Thorac Surg* 1985;39:391-399.

[4] Dahan M, Gaillard J, Eschapasse H. Surgical treatment of goiters with intrathoracic development. In: Delarue M, editor. International trends in general thoracic surgery. Vol 5. *Thoracic Surgery: frontiers and uncommon neoplasms.* St. Louis: Mosby; 1989. p. 240-246.

[5] Vadasz P, Kotsis L. Surgical aspects of 175 mediastinal goiters. *Eur J Cardiothorac Surg* 1998;14:393-397.

[6] Sancho JJ, Kraimps JL, Sanchez-Blanco JM, Larrad A, Rodríguez JM, Gil P, Gibelin H, Pereira JA, Sitges-Serra A. Increased mortality and morbidity associated with thyroidectomy for intrathoracic goiters reaching the carina tracheae. *Arch Surg* 2006;141:82-85.

[7] Allo MD, Thompson NW. Rationale for the operative management of substernal goiters. *Surgery* 1983;94:969-977.

[8] Hsu B, Reeve TS, Guinea AL, Robinson B, Delbridge L. Recurrent substernal nodule goiter: incidence and management. *Surgery* 1996;120:1072-1075.

[9] Netterville JL, Coleman SC, Smith JC, Smith MM, Day TA, Burkey BB. Management of substernal goiter. *Laryngoscope* 1998;108:1611-1617.

[10] Darwish BK, Kabbani SS. Giant substernal goiter with chylothorax. *Asian Cardiovasc Thorac Ann* 2003;11:165–166.

[11] White ML, Doherty GM, Gauger PG. Evidence-based surgical management of substernal goiter. *World J Surg* 2008;32:1285–1300.

[12] Raffaelli M, De Crea C, Ronti S, Bellantone R, Lombardi CP. Substernal goiters: incidence, surgical approach, and complications in a tertiary care referral center. *Head Neck.* 2011;33:1420-1425.

[13] Shen WT, Kepebew E, Duh QY, Clark OH. Predictors of airway complications after thyroidectomy for substernal goiter. *Arch Surg* 2004;139:656-660.

[14] Mackle T, Meaney J, Timon C. Tracheoesophageal compression associated with substernal goitre. Correlation of symptoms with cross-sectional imaging findings. *J Laryngol Otol* 2007;121:358-361.

[15] Grainger J, Saravanappa N, D'Souza A, Wilcock D, Wilson PS. The surgical approach to retrosternal goiters: the role of computerized tomography. *Otolaryngol Head Neck Surg* 2005;132:849-851.

[16] de Perrot M, Fadel E, Mercier O, Farhamand P, Fabre D, Mussot S, Dartevelle P. Surgical management of mediastinal goiters: when is a sternotomy required? *Thorac Cardiovasc Surg.* 2007;55:39-43.

[17] Newman E, Shaha AR. Substernal goiter. *J Surg Oncol* 1995;60:207-212.

[18] Hedayati N, McHenry CR. The clinical presentation and operative management of nodular and diffuse substernal thyroid disease. *Am Surg* 2002;68:245-251.

[19] Nervi M, Iacconi P, Spinelli C, Janni A, Miccoli P. Thyroid carcinoma is intrathoracic goiter. *Langenbecks Arch Surg* 1998;383:337-339.

[20] Rios A, Rodriguez JM, Balsalobre MD, Tebar FJ, Parrilla P. The value of various definitions of intrathoracic goiter for predicting intra-operative and postoperative complications. *Surgery* 2010;147:233–238.

[21] Rugiu MG, Piemonte M. Surgical approach to retrosternal goitre: do we still need sternotomy? *Acta Otorhinolaryngol Ital* 2009;29:331-338.

[22] Cohen JP. Substernal goiters and sternotomy. *Laryngoscope* 2009;119:683-688.

[23] Pieracci FM, Fahey TJ 3rd. Substernal thyroidectomy is associated with increased morbidity and mortality as compared with conventional cervical thyroidectomy. *J Am Coll Surg* 2007;205:1–7.

[24] Page C, Strunski V. Cervicothoracic goitre: an anatomical or radiological definition? Report of 223 surgical cases. *J Laryngol Otol* 2007;121:1083–1087.

[25] White ML, Doherty GM, Gauger PG. Evidence-based surgical management of substernal goiter. *World J Surg* 2008;32:1285-1300.

[26] Hashmi SM, Premachandra DJ, Bennett AMD, Parry W. Management of retrosternal goitres: results of early surgical intervention to prevent airway morbidity, and a review of the English literature. *J Laryngol Otol* 2006;120:644-649.

[27] Hedayati N, McHenry CR. The clinical presentation and operative management of nodular and diffused substernal thyroid disease. *Am Surg* 2002;68:245–252.

[28] Torre G, Borgonovo G, Amato A, Arezzo A, Ansaldo G, De Negri A, Ughè M, Mattioli F. Surgical management of substernal goiter: analysis of 237 patients. *Am Surg* 1995;61:826-831.

[29] Shaha AR. Substernal goiter: what is in a definition? *Surgery* 2010;147:239–240.

[30] Flati G, De Giacomo T, Porowska B, Flati D, Gaj F, Talarico C, Antonellis F, Diana M, Berloco PB. Surgical management of substernal goitres. When is sternotomy inevitable? *Clin Ter* 2005;156:191-195.

[31] Page C, Strunski V. Cervicothoracic goitre: an anatomical or radiological definition? Report of 223 surgical cases. *J Laryngol Otol* 2007;121:1083–1087.

[32] Rios A, Rodriguez JM, Balsalobre MD, Tebar FJ, Parrilla P. The value of various definitions of intrathoracic goiter for predicting intra-operative and postoperative complications. *Surgery* 2010;147:233–238.

[33] Pieracci FM, Fahey TJ 3rd. Substernal thyroidectomy is associated with increased morbidity and mortality as compared with conventional cervical thyroidectomy. *J Am Coll Surg* 2007;205:1–7.

[34] Sancho JJ, Kraimps JL, Sanchez-Blanco JM, Larrad A, Rodríguez JM, Gil P, Gibelin H, Pereira JA, Sitges-Serra A. Increased mortality and morbidity associated with thyroidectomy for intrathoracic goiters reaching the carina tracheae. *Arch Surg* 2006;141:82-85.

In: Thyroidectomy
Editor: Kimberly Rodolfo
ISBN: 978-1-63321-440-8

Chapter 3

Surgical Procedures and Potential Complications

Belén Pérez-Pevida[1], Cristina Zulueta Santos[2], Jimena Miranda[3] and Juan C. Galofré[1]

[1]Department of Endocrinology and Nutrition. Clinica Universidad de Navarra, Pamplona, Spain

[2]Department of Otolaryngology, Clinica Universidad de Navarra. Pamplona, Spain

[3]Department of Internal Medicine. Luis C. Lagomaggiore Hospital, Mendoza, Argentina

Abstract

Hyperthyroidism is a common condition. Its prevalence is around 2% of women and 0.2% of men [1]. Graves' disease is the most common cause of hyperthyroidism. There are three main approaches to treat hyperthyroidism: antithyroid drugs (ATD), radioiodine and surgery [2]. Surgery and radioactive iodine are two types of ablative treatments. The selection of the suitable treatment depends on a number of factors such as etiology of the dysfunction, patient's age, associated comorbidities, and potential complications [3]. Overall in Europe, ATD are usually offered whereas in the USA the first option is normally the radioiodine therapy [4,5]. Regardless of the surgical technique, any patient who is undergoing surgery should be pretreated with ATD until the patient is in euthyroid state. Thyroidectomy has suffered major changes in terms of technique and incidence of complications in the past years. Many studies in the literature correlate the complications of thyroid surgery with the surgeon's experience [6,7].

Surgical procedures: Total thyroidectomy is the recommended procedure for definitive treatment in Graves' disease, and does not increase the rate of complications compared to lobectomy in the hands of experienced surgeons. In addition, total thyroidectomy minimizes the risk of relapse. Currently there are minimally invasive techniques such as endoscopic and video-assisted thyroidectomy. These techniques have been adopted by several centers, especially in Asia and Europe. The indications include benign thyroid disease and hyperthyroidism with a relatively small thyroid volume. Endoscopic robotic thyroidectomy by axillary approach is a new technique that has some cosmetic advantages [8]. This technique offers an excellent operative field, allowing the identification of the vital structures.

Indications: Several situations such as pregnancy, reactions to ATD, rejection of radioiodine treatment, presence of Graves' ophthalmopathy, relapsed, and large goiter are some of the appropriate circumstances for surgery approach in hyperthyroidism [9-11].

Potential Complications: Thyroidectomy is associated with several complications such as: hypoparathyroidism (3.7% [0,6-50%]) [12,13], recurrent laryngeal nerve damage (1-8%) which can be transient (2.5-3% [0,9-4,7%]) [12,13] or permanent (0.3-2% [0-1,7%]) [12,13], local hemorrhage (0.36%) which can cause laryngeal edema (4.3%, [1-1,3%]) [14], thyrotoxic storm (1-2%) [15-17], surgical site infection (0,5-3%) [18-20] and recurrent hyperthyroidism (2%) [12,13].

*Conclusion:*_Although effective treatments for hyperthyroidism are available, none is perfect. Thyroid surgery is associated to negligible mortality and low complication rate [1-6]. The experience of the surgeon and the use of new, less invasive techniques, reduce the risk of postoperative complications and improve the rate of recurrence [7,8,21].

Introduction

Hyperthyroidism is a common endocrine disorder. Its prevalence is around 2% in women and 0.2% in men. Graves' disease is the most common cause of hyperthyroidism [1]. The arsenal against hyperthyroidism includes antithyroid drugs (AD), radioactive iodine therapy and surgery [2]. Around 30 to 40% of patients who are treated with antithyroid drugs remain euthyroid for prolonged time periods after the withdrawal of the drug [2]. Overall, in Europe, medical treatment is usually the first therapeutic option, whereas in the USA the first choice is commonly radioiodine [3,4]. Both surgery and radioactive iodine are two types of ablative treatment that improve thyrotoxicosis causing permanent removal or destruction of thyroid tissue [2]. This chapter is focused in the surgical approach. In order to prevent potential complications, patients who undergo surgery should be pretreated with antithyroid drugs until they achieve the euthyroid state.

In experienced hands, the rate of complications related to thyroid surgery is very low and must not exceed the 9% although they may reach 50% in some series [12, 13]. The complications that are typically associated with thyroid surgery are intraoperative and postoperative bleeding, injury of the recurrent laryngeal nerve (transient or permanent) and postoperative hypocalcaemia due to hypoparathyroidism (transient or permanent) [12-20, 22].

Preparation for Surgery

Hyperthyroid patients have to be euthyroid before the operation in order to decrease morbidity and mortality related to surgery. Thus, the first aim of pre-surgery medical treatment is the normalization of hormonal and metabolic status. These patients usually need to be treated with antithyroid drugs during several weeks, which reduces glandular thyroid hormone storage and prevents their synthesis and output [23, 24]. However, this measure does not improve the typical hyperplasia with hypervascularization of Graves' disease. For this reason some surgeons recommend pre-treatment with iodine during one week before the operation in order to reduce follicular cell size and hypervascularization. It is recommended that treatment with iodine should be initiated once the metabolic state has been normalized [23, 24].

Indication for Surgery in Hyperthyroidism

Surgical treatment in the way of thyroidectomy may be the treatment of choice in several situations such as patient preference, failed medical treatment or reactions to AD, rejection of radioiodine treatment, pregnancy, presence of Graves' ophthalmopathy, urgency of treatment (surgery is the quickest way to return a patient to the euthyroid state), relapsed hyperthyroidism or because of the presence of structural reasons. The structural conditions may comprise concomitant presence of thyroid cancer, presence of suspicious nodules with indeterminate cytology, tracheal compression, large goiter or nodule. [9-11].

> In a pregnant woman, if thyroidectomy is necessary, it should be performed during the second trimester. This should avoid the risk of miscarriage and premature delivery that may occur in the first and third trimesters, respectively [25, 26].

Surgical Procedures

Near-total or total thyroidectomy are the recommended procedures in hyperthyroidism. Well-performed thyroid surgery usually produces few complications, although total thyroidectomy is associated with a higher incidence of postoperative morbidity, this procedure minimizes the risk of relapse. Recurrence of hyperthyroidism is undesirable because a second operation is technically more difficult than the first one and involves greater risk of complications. If a second surgery is the only option, a repeat vocal cord check is mandatory and all information regarding previous surgery should be obtained. Near-total or total thyroidectomy are the recommended procedures in Graves' disease and multinodular hyperthyroidism, whereas removal of the hyperfunctioning nodule is the recommended procedure for toxic adenoma. Well-performed thyroid surgery usually produces few complications, although total thyroidectomy is associated with a higher incidence of postoperative morbidity, this procedure eliminates the risk of relapse. Recurrence of hyperthyroidism is undesirable because a second operation is technically more challenging than the first one and involves greater risk of complications. If a second surgery is the only option, a repeat vocal cord check is mandatory and all information regarding previous surgery should be obtained [27].

Standard Procedure

Usually two assistants help the surgeon. The operative table should be in a slight reverse Trendelenbourg position, which improves presentation of the operative field to the surgeon and decreases venous congestion [28].

The standard incision for thyroidectomy is the Kocher incision, placed transversely in the lower neck, at the level of the thyroid isthmus, which is situated immediately inferior to the cricoid cartilage [27]. The thyroid gland is situated underneath the infrahyoid muscles (sternohyoid and sternothyroid muscle). Once the incision is made, retraction of the skin with the platysma muscle, the subcutaneous fat and the superficial cervical fascia is needed. Then, the thyroid gland is approached by lateral retraction of the sternohyoid muscle and transection of the sternothyroid muscle [28]. The following step is the capsular dissection, i.e. the dissection between the capsula propria of the thyroid gland and the fascia covering the visceral compartment. The thyroid vessels are defined and ligated. It is critical to identify the recurrent laryngeal nerves (RLN). Systematic visualization of the RLN is the gold standard for thyroid surgery due to the decrease in RLN paralysis with this technique as compared to a 'blind' approach [29]. These nerves arise from the vagus nerve on both sides.

Thus, the right RLN recurs beneath the right subclavian artery, whereas the left recurs beneath the aortic arch. Both nerves pass posterior to the thyroid lobes and parallel the trachea as they approach the cricoid cartilage and enter the larynx. The surgical approach to finding the RLN may vary, nonetheless there are some landmarks that can help us identify the nerves: the laryngeal entry point, ligament of Berry, Tubercule of Zuckerkandl or the inferior thyroid artery. The relation between the inferior thyroid artery and the RLN may vary, hence, it is preferable to identify the inferior thyroid artery as it emerges from behind the carotid artery. Once the RLN are identified, the dissection may be completed [27].

The most common complication of total thyroidectomy is hypocalcaemia. Understanding the location and vascular anatomy of the parathyroid glands is critical to its preservation. The blood supply to the parathyroid glands is primarily from the inferior thyroid artery, though sometimes there is contribution from the superior thyroid artery. Each gland weighs 35-40 mg, measures 3-8 mm, and its color can vary from light yellow to reddish-brown [29].

The parathyroid should be dissected off the thyroid capsule and mobilized laterally with its vascular pedicle, controlling the small vessels between this capsule and the parathyroid. It is possible that the parathyroid glands are inadvertently removed during thyroidectomy; if this occurs, the parathyroid tissue may be reimplantated into an intramuscular pocket in the sternocleidomastoid muscle [27].

Minimally Invasive and Robotic Surgery

The term minimally invasive thyroid surgery encompasses a host of different techniques, which include small incision open surgery, endoscopic surgery and robotic surgery. These techniques have been developed to improve cosmetic and patient satisfaction; however, widespread adoption of these techniques cannot be recommended based on evidence [8]. A South Korean group pioneered the use of the *Da Vinci* robot (i.e. 'robotic-assisted thyroidectomy' or RT). Despite higher cost and longer operating time, it offers some advantages such as avoiding placement of cervical incision. However, RT remains controversial and specific indications are still being evaluated [8].

Various endoscopic approaches have been described, either via a lateral or central neck incision. Evidence suggests that, in the hands of experienced endoscopic endocrine surgeons, their safety outcome is comparable to open surgery, and there are obvious cosmetic advantages [21].

Potential Thyroid Surgery Complications

Overall complication rate is around 0.3-50% [12, 13]. Factors that may influence in the frequency and type of complications depend on the patient (age; presence of comorbidities such as hypertension, diabetes, heart disease); thyroid structure such as thyroid volume (hypocalcaemia rate is higher in patients with volume ≤50ml) [30]; compression of adjacent structures or infiltration of neighboring structures; clinical entity (Graves' disease or carcinoma) [1-6]. However, the main determining factors are the experience of the surgical team and the experience of the individual surgeon [6, 7].

Table 1. Potential Thyroid Surgery Complications

Complications
Recurrent hyperthyroidism
Paralysis of the vocal cords
Transient
Permanent
Hypoparathyroidism
Transient
Permanent
Hemorrhage
Wound infection

In the analysis of the study of data from patients who underwent thyroidectomy in Maryland between 1991 and 1996, individual surgeon experience, rather than hospital experience, was significantly associated with complication rates and length of stay. This relation was observed in disease and procedure subgroups, and it remained significant after adjustment for patient case mix and time period [6]. Complications are summarized in table 1.

Hypoparathyroidism

Hypoparathyroidism is the most common complication of total thyroidectomy [31-34].

The prevalence rate of thyroid surgery related hypoparathyroidism ranges between 0,6-50% with an average of 3,7%. Hypoparathyroidism can be transient (2.7%) or permanent (0.2-1.4% [12, 13]. Most cases of postoperative hypocalcaemia are clinically manifested within 72 hours after surgery.

The parathyroid glands may not be identified during surgery even after a careful capsular dissection technique because in some cases they are intrathyroidal, flattened subcapsular, hidden in the internodular grooves, or infiltrated by thyroid tumor. It is difficult to predict which patients will be at risk of unintentional parathyroid excision and whether these patients develop hypocalcemia [21, 29-32,34].

The surgical specimen of a total thyroidectomy should be examined by the surgeon after its removal to identify unintentional parathyroid gland excision. If possible parathyroid glands should be reimplantated into an intramuscular pocket in the sternocleidomastoid muscle.

Some studies have suggested measuring serum PTH levels 1 and 6 hours after the thyroidectomy. The decrease in PTH and calcium levels serves as a guide to predict the development of hypoparathyroidism. Other authors recommend a PTH cutoff level of 15 pg/mL obtained 1 hour after surgery [35, 36]. Moreover, some centers have integrated an intraoperative quick PTH assay into their practice [37].

When the parathyroid glands are injured during surgery, they may respond with complete loss of function or temporary reduction of function after minimal trauma (mainly due to ischemia) [21, 29-32].

Mild to moderate hypocalcaemia is manifested by soon paresthesia ("tingling" as reported by patients), numbness and cramps. In severe cases the alarm symptoms are carpopedal spasm, tetany crisis and impaired function of the heart muscle, with the presence of arrhythmia. On physical examination

Chvostek and Trousseau signs are present. The diagnosis is confirmed with the finding of a low blood calcium concentration [31, 32, 35]. Symptoms are relieved immediately with the intravenous administration of calcium.

Permanent hypoparathyroidism is considered when normalization of the function of the parathyroid glands is not achieved within the 6th postoperative month [31, 32, 35].

As stated earlier, there is a great variability in the literature regarding the frequency of hypoparathyroidism secondary to thyroid surgery. An estimation of the prevalence is the following:

Transient hypoparathyroidism: The prevalence ranges from 1.6 to 50% with an estimated average around 2.7% [12, 13]. The mechanisms involved include ischemia due to devascularization by ligation of vessels or secondary to vascular spasm sustained by hypothermia. Tissue warming related to light intensity (operating lights, surgeon's front light) also could be involved. Some investigators have related endothelin-1 which is an acute phase reactant that inhibits PTH secretion and has been shown to be elevated in the transient hypoparathyroidism. Other involved mechanisms may be the coexistence of hungry bone syndrome (osteodystrophy associated with hyperthyroidism), the release of calcitonin after manipulation of the gland, or decrease in serum calcium due to associated post-surgery hypoalbuminemia or hemodilution. Certainly hypomagnesemia that inhibits PTH secretion, also contributes to enhance hypocalcemic symptoms [31, 32, 35-39].

Permanent hypoparathyroidism: The prevalence ranges from 0,2 to 1.4% [12,13]. The main mechanism is the lasting gland devascularization or a direct trauma to the glands. Obviously the total removal of the parathyroid glands during surgery will head towards permanent hypocalcemia. The prevalence of unintentional parathyroidectomy during total thyroidectomy has been calculated in 12.9% [6]. The main risk factors for permanent hypocalcaemia are: female gender, small thyroid gland volume [32], elderly, reoperations, and central neck node dissection (VI area) [33-39].

The temporary parathyroid insufficiency is not a major problem, but in cases of permanent impairment, patients must carefully be reviewed and maintain a satisfactory medication indefinitely associating calcium and vitamin D to their treatment. When patients are poorly controlled, complications such as cataracts, hypertension, and nephrocalcinosis may appear.

Hypoparathyroidism occurs more frequently after thyroidectomy for Graves' disease or thyroid carcinoma. Again, it has been shown that its effect is directly related to the experience of the surgeon [6,7]. Anatomical knowledge of typical and atypical location of the four parathyroid glands, and their systematic search in any intervention, is one of the determinants of their potential damage.

Treatment: Mild hypocalcemia is treated by administration of oral calcium and vitamin D. This measure bridges the parathyroid temporary dysfunction until recovery. From the outset, it is impossible to predict whether hypoparathyroidism is transient or permanent [33, 34, 38].

The presence of symptomatic hypocalcemia is a medical emergency that requires immediate administration of intravenous calcium. Once the hypocalcaemia has been corrected treatment can be switched to oral calcium carbonate supplement at doses of 1-1.5 g every 24 h [33, 34, 38]. In the follow-up, a close monitoring of serum calcium levels is necessary. The target is to maintain serum calcium levels between 8 and 9 mg/dL [33, 34, 38].

Laryngeal Nerve Injury

> The injury of the laryngeal nerve, both of the RLN and the superior laryngeal nerve (SLN), is a typical complication of total thyroidectomy. According to different series, its frequency ranges between 1 % and 8 %. As in hypoparathyroidism, the lesion could be transient (2.5 [0,9-4,7%]) or permanent (1% [0-2%]). However, there has been a decrease in its occurrence in the last years [28].

On the other hand, the affectation could be bilateral between 0,4% and 0,9% of cases, increasing this incidence to 13% if the nerve was not identified previously; and diminishing significantly, between 0% and 6.6%, when identified previously [40,41]. The transient injury of the RLN is solved in 6 up to 8 weeks, while in permanent cases; the voice quality remains damaged, being able to improve gradually thanks to laryngeal compensation [39-42]. The unilateral damage can cause permanent hoarseness whereas the bilateral lesion drives to aphonia, hoarseness or shortness of breath that threatens patient's life. (Table 2 and 3)

RLN owes the name to its course during the embryological development. It arises from the vague nerve and appears at the end of the sixth week of the embryological development [40].

The most frequent location of the RLN is the triangle limited by the carotid sheath, the trachea and esophagus, and the low thyroid artery, being this last element its main reference. The most difficult point is when it enters into the larynx due to the close contact with the thyroid gland [39,40].

As previously mentioned, the RLN can be injured by section, traction, ischemia, compression and thermal injuries with the use of the electrosurgical unit. The surgeon's experience and anatomical knowledge represent, once more, the keystone in the injury prevention [6,7].

Table 2. Percentage of Paralysis without Previous Identification of RLN

Author	Patients (nº)	% Transient paralysis	% Permanent paralysis
Matersson y Terins [43]	514	13%	6.6%
Golliwitzer et al. [44]	1146	6%	3.8%
Pimpl et al. [45]	4154	8.7%	6.6%
Schacht et al. [46]	1274	8.5%	4.6%
Roulleau et al. [47]	987	3.5%	1%
Total	8075	7.9%	5.2%

Table 3. Percentage of Paralysis Previous Identification of RLN

Author	Patients (nº)	% Transient paralysis	% Permanent paralysis
Jacobs et al. [48]	213	0.9%	0%
Zoring et al. [49]	887	4.7%	1.4%
Ridell [50]	1700	2%	1.7%
Kark et al. [51]	325	2.2%	1.5%
Hawe y Lothian [52]	1011	2.8%	0.3%
Total	4136	2.7%	1.2%

The palsy of the RLN has an important negative impact in the patient's life, especially when it is permanent, and can be life-threatening when bilateral.

Some anomalies in the aortic arches develop a non-recurrent low laryngeal nerve. In these cases, the injury is less frequent, -between 0.3% and 0.08% on the right side, and 0,004% on the left side [39,42]. In these patients the nerve enters into the larynx at the cervical level, without descending to the thoracic level and also has been associated with a right subclavia artery that arises straight from the aortic arch. This anatomical variation is clinically important when an invasive procedure is planned in the head and neck region.

The SLN assumes less clinical importance than the RLN. Sometimes it is described as the "forgotten nerve". Nevertheless its injury has been reported even in 3.7% of total thyroidectomies, and can cause different grades of disability. It is usually located in the external face of the top constrictive muscle, although anatomical variants can exist. It has been observed that it presents a longer course in males [39-42].

The damage to this nerve can be revealed with cricothyroid muscular palsy in the ipsilateral side. Clinically the patients can warn hoarse and labored voice, throat-clearing, vocal fatigue or diminished vocal frequency, especially when raising the tone. The palsy of the SLN can be an important problem for those patients whose careers depend on the different tones of voice, such as Galli-Curci, a famous soprano that suffered this injury after a thyroid surgery with painful aftermath. To diminish its damage it is necessary to identify it and complete a precautious ligation of the top thyroid pedicle [39-42].

In cases of definitive unilateral palsy, an adaptation period is needed so that the healthy vocal cord can compensate part of the functions of the injured one, being crucial a reeducation of the voice and phoniatric rehabilitation.

The clinical manifestations also change according to the grade of affectation. If there is a unilateral palsy the vocal cord is located usually in the paramedian position and its main symptom is dysphonia. When the SLN injury is bilateral dysphonia and aspiration episodes with cough may present. In cases of bilateral palsy the vocal cords are located in median/paramedian position, developing shortness of breath. In cases of bilateral combined palsy, cords are located in intermediate or side position provoking aspirations, ineffective cough and bronchopulmonary infections [39].

Other complications exist after thyroidectomy. Most frequently changes in the tone of the voice can appear in even 42% of patients, according to the different series. These changes are due to injuries in the larynx up to 20 % of the times, more than to the damage in the nerve. Most of these take place as a result of the intubation maneuvers, provoking different dysphonia grades. Intubation and extubation may cause several injuries such as edema, granuloma, hematomas and fibrinose laryngitis or enlargement of the vocal cords [39-43].

There are other surgical risk factors associated to the injury of the RLN, many of them are related to a poor visualization of the nerve. The weight of the patient is important, since it limits the surgical collisions, as well as the presence of short necks. On the other hand, the thyroid or parathyroid surgery induces scars that modify the anatomy, and increase the risk of damaging the RLN, between 2% and 12% in a re-intervention [48]. Important tumors or very advanced grades of goiter, especially intrathoracic goiter, interfere in the identification of the nerve. Other related factors include the precedent of cervical irradiation, Graves' illness and finally thyroid gland carcinoma.

The intraoperative monitoring of the nerve is a technique that can help identify the course of the RLN and recognize its function, since the palsy might belong to a previous intervention, and this could be unknown by the patient or the doctor [53-55]. Anyhow, its use is controversial in first surgeries but some authors recognize its utility in cases of reintervention, fibrosis, aberrant path of the nerve, etc. although it neither reduces the paresis risk nor predicts the postoperative result.

Finally, regarding the treatment, a maximum period of 6 months is sufficient in order to solve injuries of neuropraxia or axonotmesis. Consequently if there is no clinical or electrophysiological evidence of recovery, a new surgery may be needed. This procedure aims to recover or to improve the voice function, to avoid the aspirations and to improve the cough reflex. In extreme cases, when damage is bilateral and the cords are in an adduction position, invasive surgeries such as tracheotomy are needed to diminish the shortness of breath [43-45]. In bilateral palsy in abduction position, tracheobronchial aspiration episodes with infections constitute the greatest problem. The ideal solution would be one that could eliminate the aspirations allowing swallowing and at the same time maintaining the phonation. Diverse treatments as the ball cannula tracheotomy have been described, and even a total laryngectomy can be necessary in case of defeat of the functional skills and bronchopulmonary severe infections. To avoid the secretions step to the trachea, laryngeal closing by occlusive laryngeal prosthesis can be practiced or even glottal suture [38-56].

Other Complications

Hemorrhage. The bleeding in the surgical field is the most serious postoperative complication. Its incidence is low, around 1-1,3% (0.36 - 4.3%) but it can be fatal if the correct diagnosis is missed [14, 56]. The suffocating hematoma causes compression and edema of pharynx and may cause choking. Intraoperative bleeding may drive to other complications due to poor identification of anatomical structures (mainly recurrent nerves and parathyroid glands) [15, 56, 57].

Bleeding is usually detected in the first 6 hours after surgery, although there have been reports of bleeding on the 5th postoperative day.

Risk factors for its presentation are high blood pressure, vomiting and Valsalva maneuvers, use of antiplatelet and anticoagulant drugs, coagulation pathology, total thyroidectomy versus lobectomy, associated lymphadenectomy, and reoperations and thyroid disease, with a higher prevalence in malignant tumors (anaplastic) and Graves' disease / hyperthyroidism [14].

As for treatment, some authors propose surgical revision if deep hematoma with stridor or hypoxia is present [56,57]. When bruising is suspected, the surgical area should be reviewed and hemostasis performed if bleeding site is located. If suffocating hematoma is presented, wound must be opened by removing the stitches immediately.

Thyrotoxic storm. It is a rare complication. Most sources report that thyroid storm accounts for between 1% and 2% of hospital admissions for thyrotoxicosis. However, some reports estimate the incidence may be as high as 10% [15-17]. It is potentially fatal and can occur intraoperatively or postoperatively. The mortality of thyroid storm is currently reported at 10% [15].

The way to avoid this complication is to preoperatively return the hyperthyroid patient to a euthyroid state. Thyroidectomy should be performed only in a euthyroidism state. Alarm symptoms should be hyperthermia, tachycardia, tremor, nausea, mental changes, and coma.

Treatment during the episode consists in immediate treatment with propylthiouracil, a beta-blocker, sodium iodide and steroids. It is necessary to start a fluid therapy replacement in order to reduce body temperature and induce diuresis. Symptomatic treatment may be progressively reduced as the patient improves along the coming weeks [15-17].

Surgical site infection. Surgical site infections (SSI) after thyroidectomy are rare but can have significant consequences. Rates of SSI in thyroidectomy are quite low, reported to be between 0.5% and 3% in most series [18-20, 22]. A deep infection may indicate pharyngeal or esophageal fistula.

Factors that increase risk of infection include immunodeficiency, diabetes and drains. Unidentified local infection may be complicated by necrotizing mediastinitis, although this is very rare [18].

Routine antibiotic prophylaxis is not recommended for clean surgical cases [18], and thyroidectomy is almost always classified as a clean case. Because of this the aseptic care during and after surgery is important in order to avoid this complication.

If signs of infection or abscess (local pain, discharge, swelling, redness) should begin, antibiotic treatment is needed, and if purulent collection is seen, drainage must be placed [18-20].

Conclusion

The management of patients with Graves' disease is controversial and continues to be debated. Although there are several treatment options, none is free of complications and the choice should be based on careful attention to the patient's clinical status and comorbidities, individualizing the characteristics and risk factors in every patient.

The goal to be achieved in the management of hyperthyroidism treatment is to reduce the secretion of thyroid hormone, achieving a euthyroid state [2]. In this chapter we have developed the indication and potential complications of total thyroidectomy for the treatment of hyperthyroidism. Surgery offers an immediate solution, eliminating the cause of hormone hypersecretion in a definitive manner, with a recurrence rate of only 2% [4, 12, 13].

Surgical treatment may be the treatment of choice in several situations such as patient preference, unsuccessful medical treatment or reactions to ATD, rejection of radioiodine treatment, pregnancy and presence of Graves' ophthalmopathy. [9-11].

The causes of postsurgical hypocalcaemia are multifactorial [4, 14, 30-34]. However, they can be avoided with a better understanding of the anatomic location of the parathyroid glands, their relationship to the recurrent laryngeal nerve and with a thorough knowledge of the surgical technique [6, 7, 29]. This also occurs with de RLN injury [40-43] hemorrhage [14, 56] and other potential complications.

Thyroidectomy should be performed only in a euthyroidism state to avoid thyrotoxic storm. [15-17].

Although the infection of the surgical wound is an uncommon process, it seems that it happens mostly in cases of thyroiditis and cancer. It is thought that both immunosuppression and longer surgeries could be risk factors. However, evidence does not recommend the use of antibiotic prophylaxis [19, 20, 22].

In summary, a complete and detailed clinical history, physical examination and laboratory and ultrasound work-out are important factors in order to predict the morbidity and possible complications of surgery [1-6]. The surgeon's experience as well as the use of modern less invasive techniques seem to be determinant factors that reduce the risk of complications [6,7], although there are only few studies concerning minimally invasive thyroid surgery.

References

[1] Stalberg P, Svensson A, Hessman O, Akerstrom G, Hellman P. Surgical treatment of graves' disease: Evidence-based approach. *World J Surg*. 2008;32(7):1269-1277.

[2] Weetman AP. Graves' disease. *N Engl J Med*. 2000;343(17):1236-1248.

[3] Harness JK, Fung L, Thompson NW, Burney RE, McLeod MK. Total thyroidectomy: Complications and technique. *World J Surg*. 1986;10(5):781-786.

[4] Prasai A, Nix PA, Aye M, Atkin S, England RJ. Total thyroidectomy for safe and definitive management of graves' disease. *J Laryngol Otol*. 2013;127(7):681-684.

[5] Patwardhan NA, Moront M, Rao S, Rossi S, Braverman LE. Surgery still has a role in graves' hyperthyroidism. *Surgery*. 1993;114(6):1108-12; discussion 1112-3.

[6] Sosa JA, Bowman HM, Tielsch JM, Powe NR, Gordon TA, Udelsman R. The importance of surgeon experience for clinical and economic outcomes from thyroidectomy. *Ann Surg*. 1998;228(3):320-330.

[7] Udelsman R. Experience counts. *Ann Surg*. 2004;240(1):26-27.

[8] Lang BH, Wong CK, Tsang JS, Wong KP, Wan KY. A systematic review and meta-analysis comparing surgically-related complications between robotic-assisted thyroidectomy and conventional open thyroidectomy. *Ann Surg Oncol*. 2014;21(3):850-861.

[9] Metso S, Jaatinen P, Huhtala H, Luukkaala T, Oksala H, Salmi J. Long-term follow-up study of radioiodine treatment of hyperthyroidism. *Clin Endocrinol (Oxf)*. 2004;61(5):641-648.

[10] Vaidya B, Williams GR, Abraham P, Pearce SH. Radioiodine treatment for benign thyroid disorders: Results of a nationwide survey of UK endocrinologists. *Clin Endocrinol (Oxf)*. 2008;68(5):814-820.

[11] Solomon B, Glinoer D, Lagasse R, Wartofsky L. Current trends in the management of graves' disease. *J Clin Endocrinol Metab*. 1990;70(6):1518-1524.

[12] Werga-Kjellman P, Zedenius J, Tallstedt L, Traisk F, Lundell G, Wallin G. Surgical treatment of hyperthyroidism: A ten-year experience. *Thyroid*. 2001;11(2):187-192.

[13] Liu Q, Djuricin G, Prinz RA. Total thyroidectomy for benign thyroid disease. *Surgery*. 1998;123(1):2-7.

[14] Spinelli C, Berti P, Miccoli P. The postoperative hemorrhagic complication in thyroid surgery. *Minerva Chir*. 1994;49(12):1245-1247.

[15] Chiha M, Samarasinghe S, Kabaker AS. Thyroid storm: An updated review. *J Intensive Care Med.* 2013.

[16] Nayak B, Burman K. Thyrotoxicosis and thyroid storm. *Endocrinol Metab Clin North Am.* 2006;35(4):663-86, vii.

[17] Wartofsky L. Thyrotoxic storm. In: *Werner and Ingbar's the thyroid.* Philadelphia: Lippincott Williams & Wilkins; 2000:679-684.

[18] Mangram AJ, Horan TC, Pearson ML, Silver LC, Jarvis WR. Guideline for prevention of surgical site infection, 1999. centers for disease control and prevention (CDC) hospital infection control practices advisory committee. *Am J Infect Control.* 1999;27(2):97-132; quiz 133-4; discussion 96.

[19] Rosato L, Avenia N, Bernante P, et al. Complications of thyroid surgery: Analysis of a multicentric study on 14,934 patients operated on in italy over 5 years. *World J Surg.* 2004;28(3):271-276.

[20] Dionigi G, Rovera F, Boni L, Castano P, Dionigi R. Surgical site infections after thyroidectomy. *Surg Infect (Larchmt).* 2006;7 Suppl 2:S117-20.

[21] Miccoli P, Materazzi G, Baggiani A, Miccoli M. Mini-invasive video-assisted surgery of the thyroid and parathyroid glands: A 2011 update. *J Endocrinol Invest.* 2011;34(6):473-480.

[22] Bergenfelz A, Jansson S, Kristoffersson A, et al. Complications to thyroid surgery: Result s as reported in a database from a multicenter audit comprising 3,660 patients. *Langenbecks Arch Surg.* 2008;393(5):667-673.

[23] Langley RW, Burch HB. Perioperative management of the thyrotoxic patient. *Endocrinol Metab Clin North Am.* 2003;32(2):519-534.

[24] Monaco F. *Thyroid diseases.* Boca Raton: Taylor & Francis; 2012.

[25] De Groot L, Abalovich M, Alexander EK, et al. Management of thyroid dysfunction during pregnancy and postpartum: An endocrine society clinical practice guideline. *J Clin Endocrinol Metab.* 2012;97(8):2543-2565.

[26] Brent GA. Clinical practice. graves' disease. *N Engl J Med.* 2008;358(24):2594-2605.

[27] Hubbard J. *Endocrine surgery: Principles and practice.* London: Springer; 2009.

[28] Gemsenjäger E. *Atlas of thyroid surgery.* Stuttgart: Thieme; 2009.

[29] Miccoli P. *Thyroid surgery: Preventing and managing complications.* Oxford: Wiley-Blackwell; 2013.

[30] Karabeyoglu M, Unal B, Dirican A, et al. The relation between preoperative ultrasonographic thyroid volume analysis and thyroidectomy complications. *Endocr Regul*. 2009;43(2):83-87.

[31] Prowse SJ, Sethi N, Ghosh S. Temporary hypocalcemia is one of the most common complications of total thyroidectomy. *Ann Otol Rhinol Laryngol*. 2012;121(12):827.

[32] Edafe O, Antakia R, Laskar N, Uttley L, Balasubramanian SP. Systematic review and meta-analysis of predictors of post-thyroidectomy hypocalcaemia. *Br J Surg*. 2014;101(4):307-320.

[33] McHenry CR, Speroff T, Wentworth D, Murphy T. Risk factors for postthyroidectomy hypocalcemia. *Surgery*. 1994;116(4):641-7; discussion 647-8.

[34] Puzziello A, Rosato L, Innaro N, et al. Hypocalcemia following thyroid surgery: Incidence and risk factors. A longitudinal multicenter study comprising 2,631 patients. *Endocrine*. 2014.

[35] Rajinikanth J, Paul MJ, Abraham DT, Ben Selvan CK, Nair A. Surgical audit of inadvertent parathyroidectomy during total thyroidectomy: Incidence, risk factors, and outcome. *Medscape J Med*. 2009;11(1):29.

[36] Richards ML, Bingener-Casey J, Pierce D, Strodel WE, Sirinek KR. Intraoperative parathyroid hormone assay: An accurate predictor of symptomatic hypocalcemia following thyroidectomy. *Arch Surg*. 2003;138(6):632-5; discussion 635-6.

[37] Wiseman JE, Mossanen M, Ituarte PH, Bath JM, Yeh MW. An algorithm informed by the parathyroid hormone level reduces hypocalcemic complications of thyroidectomy. *World J Surg*. 2010;34(3):532-537.

[38] Di Fabio F, Casella C, Bugari G, Iacobello C, Salerni B. Identification of patients at low risk for thyroidectomy-related hypocalcemia by intraoperative quick PTH. *World J Surg*. 2006;30(8):1428-1433.

[39] Herranz Gonzalez-Botas J, Lourido Piedrahita D. Hypocalcaemia after total thyroidectomy: Incidence, control and treatment. *Acta Otorrinolaringol Esp*. 2013;64(2):102-107.

[40] Mangano A, Dionigi G. The need for standardized technique in intraoperative monitoring of the external branch of the superior laryngeal nerve during thyroidectomy. *Surgery*. 2011;149(6):854-855.

[41] Rosato L, Carlevato MT, De Toma G, Avenia N. Recurrent laryngeal nerve damage and phonetic modifications after total thyroidectomy: Surgical malpractice only or predictable sequence? *World J Surg*. 2005;29(6):780-784.

[42] Sancho Fornos S, Vaqué Urbaneja J, Ponce Marco J, Palasí Giménez R, Herrera Vela C. Complicaciones de la cirugía tiroidea. *Cir Esp.* 2001;69(03):198-203; 203.

[43] Martensson H, Terins J. Recurrent laryngeal nerve palsy in thyroid gland surgery related to operations and nerves at risk. *Arch Surg.* 1985;120(4):475-477.

[44] Gollwitzer M, Mattes P, Nagel B. The spontaneous regression of recurrent nerve paralysis after goiter surgery. *Med Welt.* 1982;33(5):172-174.

[45] Pimpl W, Gruber W, Steiner H. Course of recurrent nerve paralysis after thyroid operation. *Chirurg.* 1982;53(8):505-507.

[46] Schacht U, Kremer K, Gross M, Versmold W. Incidence of latent and manifest recurrent paralysis following thyroid operations. *Zentralbl Chir.* 1972;97(44):1578-1583.

[47] Roulleau P, Blondeau P, Trotoux J. Recurrent nerve risk in thyroid surgery. (study of a series of 1,000 operations). *Ann Otolaryngol Chir Cervicofac.* 1973;90(9):519-525.

[48] Jacobs JK, Aland JW,Jr, Ballinger JF. Total thyroidectomy. A review of 213 patients. *Ann Surg.* 1983;197(5):542-549.

[49] Zornig C, de Heer K, Koenecke S, Engel U, Bay V. Identification of the recurrent laryngeal nerve in thyroid gland surgery--a status determination. *Chirurg.* 1989;60(1):44-48.

[50] Riddell V. Thyroidectomy: Prevention of bilateral recurrent nerve palsy. results of identification of the nerve over 23 consecutive years (1946-69) with a description of an additional safety measure. *Br J Surg.* 1970;57(1):1-11.

[51] Kark AE, Kissin MW, Auerbach R, Meikle M. Voice changes after thyroidectomy: Role of the external laryngeal nerve. *Br Med J (Clin Res Ed).* 1984;289(6456):1412-1415.

[52] Hawe P, Lothian KR. Recurrent laryngeal nerve injury during thyroidectomy. *Surg Gynecol Obstet.* 1960;110:488-494.

[53] Eisele D, Smith R. *Complications in head and neck surgery.* Edinburgh: Saunders; 2008.

[54] Chuang YC, Huang SM. Protective effect of intraoperative nerve monitoring against recurrent laryngeal nerve injury during re-exploration of the thyroid. *World J Surg Oncol.* 2013;11:94-7819-11-94.

[55] Postma GN, Blalock PD, Koufman JA. Bilateral medialization laryngoplasty. *Laryngoscope.* 1998;108(10):1429-1434.

[56] Lee HS, Lee BJ, Kim SW, et al. Patterns of post-thyroidectomy hemorrhage. *Clin Exp Otorhinolaryngol*. 2009;2(2):72-77.

[57] Rosenbaum MA, Haridas M, McHenry CR. Life-threatening neck hematoma complicating thyroid and parathyroid surgery. *Am J Surg*. 2008;195(3):339-43; discussion 343.

In: Thyroidectomy
Editor: Kimberly Rodolfo

ISBN: 978-1-63321-440-8

Chapter 4

Thyroid Surgery Complications

***Pietro Iacconi*[1*], *Marco Puccini*[1†]**
and Gianluca Donatini*[2], *MD, PhD, FEBS
[1]Associate professor of Surgery, Pisa University, Italy
[2](Endocrine Surgery) CHU Poitiers, Poitiers, France

Abstract

Thyroidectomy is a well standardized procedure. Currently mortality rate is reduced close to zero and its complications are not worrisome. Technical progress and wide attention to the cosmetic results have pushed the development of new surgical techniques, namely Minimal Invasive Video Assisted thyroidectomy (MIVAT) and transaxillary robotic thyroidectomy. MIVAT can be considered a miniaturization of traditional cervicotomic approach with a similar spectrum of complications. In the literature have been described a subcutaneous reimplant from a benign goiter. With the transaxillary approach the spectrum of complications have been broadened with tunnel associated problems and the position of the arm. One of the authors (MP) have observed a neoplastic reimplant in the tunnel. The main complications of the classic thyroidectomy are:

- Acute post-operative hemorrage with compressive hematoma: this causes asphyxia, that requests emergency decompression.

* pietro.iacconi@gmail.com.
† marco.puccini@med.unipi.it.

When bleeding is less dramatic we observe a subcutaneous hematoma, which determines a visible lump without respiratory problems

- Hypocalcemia is routinely checked and can be symptomatic or a laboratory diagnosis, associated with overt symptoms or not. The asymptomatic one can be a mild form of hypo-parathyroidism, deserving some forms of treatment or can reflect a low protein level: this does not deserve any treatment.
- Recurrent laryngeal nerve injury can be transient or permanent, unilateral or bilateral: the last is one of the most dramatic acute event in thyroid surgery. In the recent years many surgeons have suggested the use of neuromonitoring (NIM) to reduce the incidence of nerve palsy and more to avoid bilateral palsy with a staged thyroidectomy.

Other complication of thyroid surgery are:

- wound problems, like seroma, infection, cutaneous sensitive neck problems and a bad scar
- swallowing disorders
- chilous fistula
- Horner syndrome
- tracheal or esophageal injury

Further peculiar complications are associated to the dissection of lateral compartment of the neck.

Introduction

Mortality for thyroid surgery, in our era is virtually absent. In the eighteenth century mortality was 40% due to bleeding and sepsis. [1]

Systematic haemostasis allowed Kocher to lower mortality from 15% to 2,4% and in 1898 he published a paper reporting an overall incidence of mortality for thyroidectomy of 0,18%.

Afterword the complications came in evidence. Today surgeons are concerned by the three major complications: hypo-parathyroidism, recurrent nerve palsy and post-operative bleeding. Sosa [2] demonstrated that there is a relevant inverse relationship between the number of operations performed by any surgeon and the occurrence of complications. Apart from surgical complication there are also a 1,5% of non-surgical complications reported: respiratory, urological, gastrointestinal, cardiac and drug allergies. Notoriously it's really difficult to get an actual percentage of complications in thyroid surgery because almost always their incidence is underreported [3].

Major complications (hypoparathyroidism and laryngeal nerve palsy) cause a life-long impairment and reduced life quality to patient, while post-operative bleeding may be life-treathening.

Patient's Position

Anaesthetist and the surgeon are in charge for the correct position of the patient on the table. Cervical and Brachial plexus and the ulnar nerve are at the risk, during patient installation. It should be avoided head's hyperextension in patients with cervical disc hernia. Moreover head hyperextension causes cephalea in the post-operative period.

Laryngeal Nerve Palsy

Recurrent laryngeal nerve damage is the most frequent malpractice litigation.

Any surgeon knows the anatomic variations of the nerve (recurrent not recurrent, more branches). Classically we are teached where to watch for finding the nerve: its crossing with the carotid artery, with inferior thyroid artery, at Berry ligament [4]. Today watching for the nerve is considered mandatory [2, 4, 5, 6, 7, 8, 9].

The inferior laryngeal nerve may be harmed by multiple actions: cutting, clamping, tractioning, compression (by instruments, oedema or hematoma) and thermal injury by electro coagulation. The damage can be transient or permanent (when the nerve does not recovers after 6-12 months). Rarely the damage is recognized during the operation: on occasion we advice to try a primary repair using microsurgical techniques with epineural sutures. When a long tract of the nerve is lacking the great auricular nerve can be interposed. The resumption of function is rarely obtained, but primary reconstruction can improve vocal cord function [10]. The late reconstruction has a minor possibility of success.

When the vocal cord remains in a para-median position usually the patient is asymptomatic. That is why an ORL exam is always requested before and after the operation [9]. If the vocal cord remains in a lateral position, the patients are dysphonic (hoarseness and aspiration). These subjects request logopedia and eventually injection or medialization laryngoplasty.

Many monitoring methods are suggested to preserve the functional more than anatomical nerve integrity. Neuromonitoring is currently under development and is claimed to be more efficient than simple intraoperative visual inspection, and also to represent a better instrument in case of medico-legal litigation [12, 13, 14]. There are some controversies about: the risk probably is not reduced and this outcome can not be predicted [11].

A bilateral recurrent laryngeal nerve injury implies a median vocal cord position with airway obstruction. Rosato [14] reports his frequency as high as 0,4% of all thyroidectomies. At awakening the acute respiratory distress requests immediate re-intubation and high doses of cortisone. Extubation is attempted after 24-72 hours in a safe environment (possibly ICU or in OR, with the chance of an emergency tracheostomy).

Extubation is usually successful if the nerve palsy is temporary. If respiratory distress persists orotracheal intubation is mandatory and tracheostomy (either transient or definitive) must be considered. It is usually definitive if after 9-12 months a bilateral vocal cords palsy is still present. Alternatively a cordotomy may be performed. [15].

Due to the risk of bilateral palsy and that may be a difficult reintubation, we leave the operating table sterile till the complete awakening of the patients (estubation): when the patient breathes normally and surely is not bleeding.

The modern *energy based devices* (Ligasure, Ultracision) inspire confidence: this induces to neglect that like the normal monopolar electrocautery generate heat, with the risk of damaging the nerve [16, 17].

As a matter of principle we do not use sources of energy in proximity of the nerve. We suggest bipolar coagulation at a very low power, using a sharp points device and with bursts not longer than 1-2 seconds.

Diagnosis of a lesion of the external branch of the superior laryngeal nerve (EBSLN) is more difficult. Recently IONM has been used successfully for the identification of the EBSLN [18]. Although its damage does not determine respiratory distress it may be extremely harmful for professional voice users (teachers, singers….). To reduce the risk of a EBSLN Lenquist suggests a super-selective ligation of the superior vascular pole, because often this branch intermingles the upper pole pedicle [19] Careful use of energy based devices as well electrocautery at this level is also requested. By notice about 0,3% of the laryngeal damages reported are due to the orotracheal intubation [20].

Post-Operative Bleeding

Post-operative bleeding is a potentially lethal complication. It is heralded by respiratory distress, cervical oppression and voice changes [14].

Bleeding usually occurs in the first 12 post-operative hours. This is the main reason why most endocrine surgeons avoid thyroidectomy as an outpatients procedure [21, 22]. In the presence of a neck hematoma, the wound must be re-opened to avoid dead by asphyxiation. It may be sometimes required directly at the bed of the patient (in the ward or recovery room). It is not necessary (there is not time) any local anaesthesia.

At the end of surgery we routinely verify the haemostasis using some tricks: the patient is either moved in a Trendelemburg position or we ask the anaesthesiologist to perform a Valsalva manoever. Routine use of drainage does not avoid bleeding neither surely consent a hematoma diagnosis. We must consider that anaesthesiologist may have difficulty in achieve an oro-tracheal intubation in case of compressive neck hematoma. A set for tracheostomy and a set with few sterile instruments (forceps, scissors, Kelly clamps) must be available in the ward. Usually the evacuation of the hematoma is sufficient to decompress the trachea and to allow intubation. Remarkably, in our experience, cervical exploration in a patient with a post-operative neck hematoma rarely identifies a sure source of bleeding. The new techniques of minimal access thyroidectomy, both cervical and extracervical, seem to have the same incidence of postoperative bleeding, according to the systematic review of Chen [23]. Avoiding postoperative nausea and vomiting could reduce the risk of post-operative bleeding; so many surgical teams adopt postoperative nausea and vomiting (PONV) protocols.

Hypocalcemia

Hypocalcemia is reported in the literature in a percentage between 1 and 50%. [24]

In a recent review [25] the median incidence of transient and permanent hypocalcemia was 27 [19-38] and 1 (0-3) percent respectively.

Postoperative hypocalcemia is multifactorial [25, 26].

It can be due to unintentional removal of the parathyroids or their devascularisation. Knowledge of their anatomy and vascular supply is mandatory for their salvage.

To maintain a sufficient blood flow to the parathyroids is essential to perform selective ligations of the branches of inferior thyroid artery (ITA) and to avoid an en-bloc ligation of it. Remarkably 20% of vascularization of the inferior parathyroid gland may belong from branches of the superior vascular pedicle, but mostly it comes from ITA and sometimes from subcapsular thyroid branches.

There is no agreement in the literature about how many parathyroids are needed to achieve eucalcemia. Some authors sustain that just one vital parathyroid gland is enough while some others stand for at least three [27].

If a gland looks ischemic or is not possible to be left in place correctly vascularised it must be transplanted. Usually this is performed creating a pouch in the sternocleidomastoid muscle; the site of transplantation is often marked by not resorbable stich or metallic clips. Biopsy of normal glands must be avoided [28].

The prophylactic dissection of the central compartment of the neck is a procedure associated to an increase in the incidence of postoperative hypocalcemia, due to an extensive manipulation of the parathyroid glands, especially the lower ones. And transient hypocalcemia seems to be the most important complication with central neck dissection. If it is excluded, then a thyroidectomy with central dissection has the same morbidity of a total thyroidectomy alone [29, 30].

Calcemia is routinely measured during the postoperative course. Patient with symptomatic hypocalcemia are treated by the administration of calcium and vitamin D derivatives. Patients with asymptomatic hypocalcemia are managed with different strategies by surgeons. Each professional tries to develop a local management protocol, so "biochemical" hypoparathyroidism represents a very controversial issue. According to some authors the measurement of parathormone levels (PTH) could allow a safely early discharge [31]. Half-life of PTH is around 5', so then a PTH measurement late after the surgery (6 h to 24h) may allow recognizing surgical hypoparathyroidism. Other Authors combine the measurement of PTH and calcium to institute a supplemental treatment [32].

Hypocalcemia is managed by calcium carbonate (2-8 grams per die) and Vit D supplementation. In case of symptomatic hypocalcemia (ranging from peripheral numbness to titanic crisis) intravenous administration of calcium gluconate may ameliorate these symptoms. To prevent post-thyroidectomy hypocalcemia and to avoid the experience of hypocalemia symptoms, many authors suggest the prophylactic administration of calcium and/or vitamin D derivatives. A systematic review on this topic has been recently published, that recommend oral calcium for all patients following thyroidectomy, with the addition of vitamin D for high-risk individuals [33, 34]. Nevertheless, usually the administration of calcium and vitamin D supplementation is made on the basis of some measurable variable, usually calcium levels on postoperative day 1 and 2. Many examples are available in the literature [35].

In the literature there is a wide range of definition and a lack of consensus on the definition of hypocalcemia [36]. It may be transient or definitive. Usually transient hypocalcemia lasts less than 6 months, while after 6 months it is considered definitive. This is associated with a significant impairment of quality of life. At the moment the transplantation of parathyroid is not available [37].

Chylous Fistula

Toracic duct lesion may occur during left lateral neck dissection. If recognized intraoperatively must be immediately stopped by suturing or tying. When the diagnosis is made postoperatively, there are two options, depending from the load of the chylous fistula. If the 24 hours amount is less than 400 ml it can be managed conservatively by fasting, total parenteral nutrition [38]. Short chain fatty acid can be useful. Somatostatin use has been reported. For high output fistulas (more than 400 ml/24 h) management require an invasive procedure (early surgical closure of the fistula or percutaneous radiological intervention [39, 40]. Administration of a fat-rich meal (e.g. ice-cream with high content of butter) 3-4 hours before the operation allows a prompt recognition of a leak, due to the chylomicron-rich lymph which is easily visible (Figures 1, 2).

Scar and Wound Infections

Wound healing usually is not remarkable. Nevertheless all the principles of plastic surgery should be respected. For example one of the most common mistakes is to perform a small incision then stretch skin and subcutaneous tissues by over-traction to achieve a larger operatory field [41]. Another important aspect regards the neck incision. It has to be made at least 2 cm above the sternal notch. The closest the incision stands to the presternal aera the highest is the risk of a cheloid development. Moreover there are racial differences in wound healing. Usually Caucasians and Asiatics show a minor predisposition to cheloid development than Afroamericans (Fig 3).

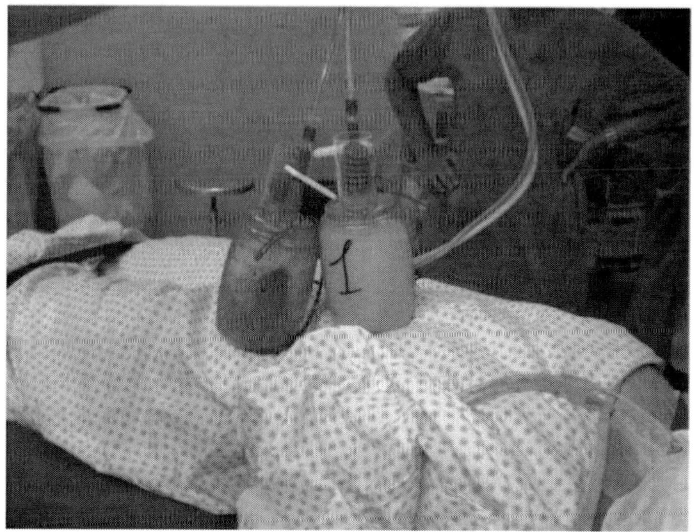

Figure 1. Typical chylous content in the drain.

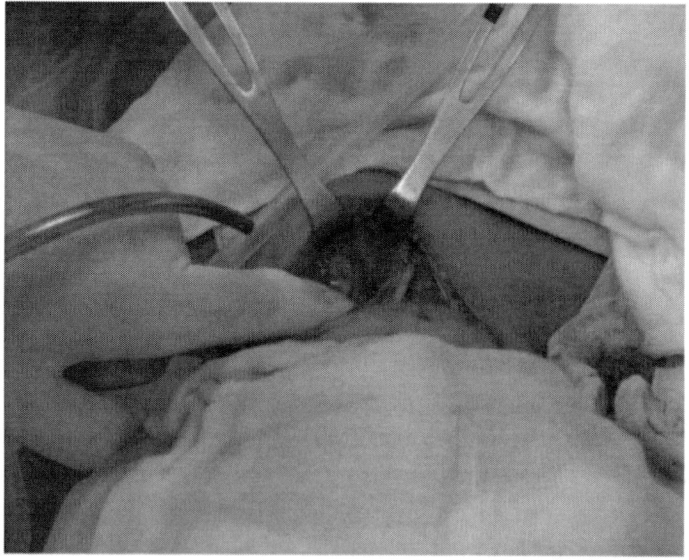

Figure 2. Operative findings. Chylous secretion within operative field.

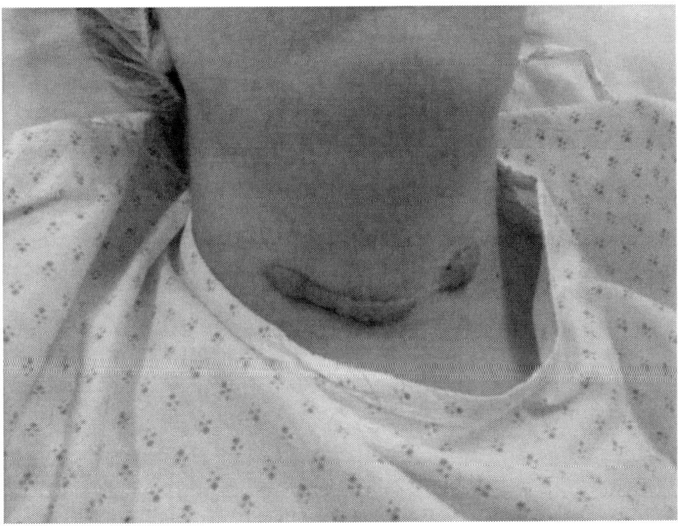

Figure 3. Cheloid scar along the neck incision in a young north-African lady.

Wound infections, usually due to staphilococci and/or streptococci, are reported in between 0,3% and 0,8%[2]. Routinary use of antibiotics is not indicated except in immuno-compromized subjects and for patients with previous cardiac surgery or valvulopathies. When present an abscess must be immediately drained for the risk of mediastinitis. Seromas may be managed conservatively or by needle aspiration.

Tracheal Instability

Tracheomalacia is described, in many textbooks, as a potential occurrence in long-term big goitres. It is a real rare finding and, if suspected, endoluminal stenting has been suggested in order to gain tracheal stability. Personally in doubt of tracheomalacia I have put two stitches, one on each side of the trachea; the extremes of the threads were left free outside of the skin. These, in the case of necessity, can be tied on a swab roll to maintain open the trachea. They can be used for make an emergency tracheostomy. Some days after we can cut the treads outside of the skin. Tracheotomy is the last option for tracheomalacia.

Rare Complications

Among rare complications, some neural, vascular and visceral lesions are reported [29]. Cervical sympathetic chain damage is reported in one of 5000 operations, especially in retro-esophageal goitres [24]. Its damage causes a Bernard Horner syndrome. Phrenic and the accessory spinal nerve are more at risk during lateral neck dissection. A lesion of these nerves is responsible, respectively, of an elevation of the hemidiaphragm and a drop of the shoulder with difficulty in his elevation.

Pneumothorax or laceration of the subclavian artery or vein is described for large substernal goitres. Overtraction on an atherosclerotic carotid may determine an occlusion of its lumen or damage to its wall, so causing a neurological damage due to blood flow alteration (either ischemia or reperfusion edema).

A lesion of the oesophageal wall is rare. Immediate suture of the leak, positioning of a nasogastric tube, fasting with total intravenous nutrition is mandatory.

Tracheal laccration is very rare: Gosnell JE et al. have described the mechanism of injury [43,44].

Thyroid storm is today an exceptional evenience. Tachycardia, nausea and vomiting, restlessness, mental alteration and even coma are the typical signs and symptoms. Patients, especially with hyperthyroidism, should be managed pre-operatively with anti-thyroid drugs, beta-blockers and iodine to avoid this complication.

New Techniques

The last evolution of approaches to the thyroid gland consists of robotic approaches. According to first reports, it seems to be no difference about the complications rate with respect to conventional approach, the advantage of axillary approaches consisting in cosmetic satisfaction score. Robotic trans-axyllary approaches may introduce the risk of new complications (tunnel related complications, inadvertent implantation of thyroid tissue) and require longer operative times. Furthermore, the positioning of the patient raises the risk of brachial plexus injury [45, 46, 47].

As far as minimally invasive, video-assisted approach (MIVAT) the meta-analysis of available randomized clinical trials comparing MIVAT versus conventional thyroidectomy shows no important differences in the incidence / quality of complications, but just a longer operative time associated to the minimally invasive approach, counterbalanced by a better cosmetic score and less postoperative pain [48, 49].

References

[1] Becker WF, Pioneers in thyroid surgery. *Ann Surg* 185:493-504 (1977).

[2] Sosa JA, Bowman HM, Gordon TA, Bass EB, Yeo CJ, Lillemoe KD, Pitt HA, Tielsch JM, Cameron JL, The importance of surgeon experience for clinical and economic outcomes from thyroidectomy. *Ann Surg* 228: 320-330 (1998).

[3] Dickersin K, The existence of pubblication bias and risk factors for its occurrence. *JAMA* 263:1385-1389 (1990).

[4] Randolph GW, Surgical anatomy of the recurrent laryngeal nerve. Chapter 33, pag 306-340 in Surgery of the thyroid and parathyroid glands, Gregory W Randolph, second edition. *Elsevier Saunders* 2013.

[5] Herman M et al, Laryngeal recurrent nerve injury in surgery for benign thyroid diseases: effect of nerve dissection and impact of individual surgelo in more than 27.000 nerves at risk. *Ann Surg* 235:251-268 (2002).

[6] Jatzko GR, Lisborg PH, Muller MG, Wette VM, Recurrent nerve palsy after thyroid operations: principal nerve identification and a literature review. *Surgery* 115: 139-144 (1994).

[7] Wagner HE, Seiler C, Recurrent laringea nerve palsy after thyroid gland surgery. Br J Surg 81:226-228 (1994).

[8] Goncalves Filho J, Kolwalski LP, Surgical complications after thyroid surgery performer in arance hospital. *Otorinolaryngol Head Neck Surg* 132:490-494.

[9] Steurer M et al. Advantages of recurrent laringeal nerve identification in thyroidectomy and parathyroidectomy and the importance of preoperative and postoperative laryngoscopic examination in more than 1000 nerves at risk. *Laryngoscope* 112:124-133 (2002).

[10] Simon D, Lassau M, Schmidt-Wilcke P, Boucher M.: Intraoperative complications of neck surgery. *Chirurg;* 83(7):626-32 (2012).

[11] Beldi G, Kinsbergen T, Schlumpf R Evaluation of intraoperative recurrent nerve monitoring in thyroid surgery. *World J Surg* 28:589-591 (2004).

[12] Dralle H, Sekulla C, Haerting J, Timmerman W, et al, Risk factors of paralysis and functional out come after recurrent laryngeal nerve monitoring in thyroid surgery. *Surgery* 136:1310-1322 (2004).

[13] Domoslawski P, Lukienczuk T, Kaliszewski K, Sutkowski K, Wojczys R, Wojtczak B.: Safety and current achievements in thyroid surgery with neuromonitoring. *Adv Clin Exp Med.* 22(1):125-30 (2013).

[14] Rosato L, Avenia N, Bernante P, De Palma M, Gulino G, Nasi PG, Pelizzo MR, Pezzullo L. Complications of thyroid surgery: analysis of a multicentric study on 14934 patients operated on in Italy over 5 years. *World J Surg* 28: 271-276 (2004).

[15] Fewins J, SimpsonCB, Miller FR Complications of thyroid and parathyroid surgery. *Otolaryngol Clin N Am* 36: 189-206 (2003).

[16] Agarwal BB, Agarwal S Rercurrent laringea nerve, phonation and voice preservation- Energy devices in thyroid surgery- a note of caution. *Langenbeck Arch Surg* 394: 911-912 (2009).

[17] Dionigi G Reply to dR Agarwal's letter to editor"Recurrent laringea nerve, phonation and voice preservation –energy devices in thyroid surgery- anote of caution. *Arch Surg* 394: 913-914 (2009).

[18] Barczynski M, Randolph GW, Cernea CR, Dralle H, Dionigi G, Alesina PF, Mihai R, Finck C, Lombardi D, Hartl DM, Miyauchi A, Serpell J, Snyder S, Volpi E, Woodson G Kraimps JL, Hisham. AN External branch of the superior laringea nerve monitoring during thyroid and parathyroid surgery: International Neural Monitoring Study Group standars guideline statement. *Laryngoscope.*

[19] Lenquist S, Cahliu C, Smeds S. The superior laringeal nerve in thyroid surgery *Surgery* 102(6): 999-108 (1987).

[20] Peppard SB, Dickens JH Laryngeal injury following short-term intubation. *Ann Otol Rhinol Laryngol* 92:327-330 (1983).

[21] Menegaux F Ambulatory thyroidectomy: recommendations from Association Francophone de Chirurgie Endocrinienne (AFCE), *J Visc Surg* 150(3): 165-171 (2013).

[22] Rutledge J, Siegel E, Belcher R, Bodenner D, Stack BC, Barriers to same day discharge of patients undergoing total and completion thyroidectomy. *Otolaryngol Head Neck Surg* 150 (5): 770-4 (2014)

[23] Chen GZ, Zhang X, ShiWL, Zhuang ZR, Chen X, Han H: Systematic comparison of cervical and extracervical surgical approaches for endoscopic thyroidectomy. *Surg Today* 42 (9): 835-841 (2012).

[24] Reeve T, Thompson NW Complications of thyroid surgery: how to avoid them, how to manage them and observations of their possible effect on the whole patient. *World J Surg* 24:971-975 (2000).

[25] Edafe O, Prasad P, Harrison BJ, Balasubramanian SP Incidence and predictors of post-thyroidectomy hypocalcemia in a tertiary endocrine surgical unit. *Ann R Coll Surg Engl* 96 (3): 219-223 (2014).

[26] McHenry CR, Speroff T, Wentworth D, Murphy T, Risk factors for postthyroidectomy hypocalcemia. *Surgery* 116:641-648 (1994).

[27] Pattou F, Combemale F, Fabre S, Carnaille B, Decoulx M, Wemeau Jl, Racadot A, Proye C, Hypocalcemia following thyroid surgery: incidence and prediction of out come. *World J Surg* 22:718-724 (1998).

[28] Olson JA, DeBenedetti MK, Baumann DS, Wells SA, Parathyroid autotranspalntation during thyroidectomy. Results of long-term follow-up. *Ann Surg* 223:472-480 (1996).

[29] Lang 2013, Lang BH, Ng SH, Lau LL, Cowling BJ, Wong KP, Wan KY: A systematic review and meta-analysis of prophylactic central neck dissection on short-term locoregional recurrence in papillary thyroid carcinoma after total thyroidectomy. *Thyroid.* 2013 Sep;23(9):1087-98

[30] Giordano 2012 Giordano D, Valcavi R, Thompson GB, Pedroni C, Renna L, Gradoni P, Barbieri V.: Complications of central neck dissection in patients with papillary thyroid carcinoma: results of a study on 1087 patients and review of the literature. *Thyroid.* 22(9):911-7 (2012).

[31] Quiros RM et al. Intraoperative parathyroid hormone levels in thyroid surgery are predictive of postoperative hypoparathyroidism and need for vitamin D supplementation. *Am J Surg* 189: 306-309 (2005).

[32] Lombardi CP, Raffaelli M, Princi P, Santini S, Boscherini M, De Crea C, Traini E, D'Amore AM, Carrozza C, Zuppi C, Bellantone R, Early prediction of postoperative hypocalcemia by one single iPTH measurement, *Surgery* 136(6): 1236-41 (2004).

[33] Alhefdhi A, Mazeh H, Chen H.: Role of postoperative vitamin D and/or calcium routine supplementation in preventing hypocalcemia after thyroidectomy: a systematic review and meta-analysis. *Oncologist* 18(5): 533-42 (2013).

[34] Wang TS, Roman SA, Sosa JA: Postoperative calcium supplementation in patients undergoing thyroidectomy. *Curr Opin Oncol.* 24(1): 22-8 (2012).

[35] Landry CS, Grubbs EG, Hernandez M, Hu MI, Hansen MO, Lee JE, Perrier ND: Predictable criteria for selective, rather than routine,

calcium supplementation following thyroidectomy. *Arch Surg.* 147(4): 338-44 (2012).

[36] Mehanna HM, Jain A, Randeva H, Watkinson J, Shaha A: Postoperative Hypocalcemia- the differernce a decision makes, *Head Neck* 32:279-283 (2010).

[37] Hasse C et al. Parathyroid xenotransplantation without immunosuppression in experimental hypoparathyroidism: long-term in vivo function following microencapsulation with clinically suitable alginate. *World J Surg* 24: 1361-1366 (2000).

[38] Lopez Otero MJ, Fernandez lopez MT, Outeirino Blanco E, Alvarez Vazquez P: Fistula linfatica cervical: manejo conservador *Nutr Hosp* 25(6): 1041-1044 (2010)

[39] Ikeda Y: Thoracoscopic management of cervical thoracic duct injuries after thyroidectomy with lymphadenectomy *Asian J Endosc Surg* 7(1): 82-84 (2014).

[40] Cope C Management of unremitting chilothorax by percutaneous embolization, *J Vasc Interv Radiol* 13(11): 1139-48 (2002).

[41] Brunaud L, Zarnegar R, Wade N, Ituarte P, Clock OH, Duh QY, Incision lengh for standard thyroidectomy and parathyroidectomy: when is it minimally invasive?, *Arch Surg* 138(10):1140-3 (2003).

[42] ReeveT, Thompson NW, Complications of thyroid surgery: how to avoid them, how to manage them, and observations on their possible effect on whole patient. *World J Surg* 24(8): 971-5 (2000).

[43] Gosnell JE, Campbell P, Sidhu S, Reeve TS, Delbridge LW, Inadvertent tracheal perforation during thyroidectomy; *Br J Surg* 93(1): 55-56 (2006).

[44] Iacconi P. Comment on Inadvertent tracheal perforation Br J Surg. 2006.

[45] Sun GH, Peress L, Pynnonen MA: Systematic Review and Meta-analysis of Robotic vs conventional Thyroidectomy Approaches for Thyroid Disease. *Otolaryngol Head Neck Surg.* 2014 Feb 5. [Epub ahead of print].

[46] Lang BH, Wong CK, Tsang JS, Wong KP, Wan KY: A Systematic Review and Meta-analysis Comparing Surgically-Related Complications between Robotic-Assisted Thyroidectomy and Conventional Open Thyroidectomy. *Ann Surg Oncol.* 21(3): 850-61 (2014).

[47] Luginbuhl A, Schwartz DM, Sestokas AK, Cognetti D, Pribitkin E.: Detection of evolving injury to the brachial plexus during transaxillary robotic thyroidectomy. *Laryngoscope*. 122(1): 110-5 (2012).

[48] Pisanu A, Podda M, Reccia I, Porceddu G, Uccheddu A: Systematic review with meta-analysis of prospective randomized trials comparing minimally invasive video-assisted thyroidectomy (MIVAT) and conventional thyroidectomy (CT). *Langenbecks Arch Surg*. 398(8): 1057-68 (2013).

[49] Radford PD, Ferguson MS, Magill JC, Karthikesalingham AP, Alusi G.: Meta-analysis of minimally invasive video-assisted thyroidectomy. *Laryngoscope*. 121(8): 1675-81 (2011).

In: Thyroidectomy
Editor: Kimberly Rodolfo
ISBN: 978-1-63321-440-8

Chapter 5

Thyroidectomy: Indications, Technique and Perioperative Care

***Dilip Dan*[1], *Kavita Deonarine*[2], *Christian Beharry*[2], *Shamir Cawich*[1] *and Vijay Naraynsingh*[1]**

[1]Department of Clinical Surgical Sciences, Faculty of Medical Sciences, University of the West Indies St. Augustine Campus, St. Augustine, Trinidad and Tobago, West Indies

[2]Residents Faculty of Medical Sciences, University of the West Indies St. Augustine Campus, St. Augustine, Trinidad and Tobago, West Indies

Abstract

The first thyroidectomy was performed in Baghdad circa 500 BC, but it was not until Emile Theodor Kocher refined his operative technique in the nineteenth century that it became accepted as a mainstream operative procedure. Due to the intricate relationship of numerous important functional structures in the neck, thyroidectomy was still fraught with life altering, and sometimes life threatening, complications. Despite this, surgical intervention for thyroid disease remains as one of the pillars of treatment with 80,000 thyroidectomies being performed in the United States annually [1].

We reviewed the surgical anatomy of the thyroid gland along with its relations to the parathyroid glands, recurrent and external laryngeal

nerves in a prior chapter in this book. Anatomic variations were discussed as well as tips and tricks to identify these important structures at the time of surgery.

The indications for thyroidectomy together with the necessary pre-operative assessment including history, examination, thyroid function tests, ultrasound and fine needle aspiration cytology will be reviewed. The role of Computerised Tomography scan, radionucleotide scanning and Magnetic Resonance Imaging will be mentioned.

Traditional thyroid surgery involved the use of cold steel. In this era, bleeding was a major concern as the vessels are numerous and thin walled and they may retract to make control difficult. With the introduction of monopolar and bipolar diathermy operative time has decreased. Operative time and blood loss are even shorter now with the use of ultrasonic dissectors [2]. Other tools including nerve stimulators will be discussed and the data analysed.

Recent advances in surgical equipment has fostered an evolution of the traditional thyroidectomy technique using sub-platysmal flaps. Considering that cosmesis remains one of the main indications for this operation, we have witnessed the introduction of video assisted thyroidectomy and robotic thyroidectomy. These minimally invasive techniques are explored, including their cost-benefit ratios and learning curves.

We also discuss modifications of the traditional open technique including the retrograde sub-capsular approach that facilitates preservation of the external branch of the superior laryngeal nerve when removing large bulky glands. We also strive to discuss means to prevent complications, treat them and look at the long term outcomes.

A Brief History of Surgery of the Thyroid Gland

The history of thyroid surgery dates back thousands of years. A rudimentary understanding of the thyroid gland as an endocrine organ existed with goiters being recognized by the Chinese in 2700 B.C. and the Indian Ayurvedic system as 'Gala Ganda' in 1400 BC [3].

Details of the thyroid gland first appeared in the drawings of Da Vinci in 1511 with detailed anatomy being described by Andreas Vesalius (1514–1564). Eustachius (1520–1547) described the isthmus and the term thyroid was coined by Thomas Warton. James Berry described the ligamentum thyroideum in the 1800's [4].

The genesis of thyroid surgery has deep historical roots with the first thyroidectomy being performed in Baghdad around 500 BC followed by work in the first and second century by Celsus and Galen [2]. Research continued in Europe with Lorenz Heister describing colloid substance in 1754 and acknowledging that goiters can become malignant. Further interest in thyroid function continued with Kocher performing 2000 thyroid excisions by 1912, the first being in 1876 [5].

Despite continuing research and development of new techniques thyroid surgery even in the hands of experienced surgeons was a life threatening procedure in the 1800's. Kocher saw a decrease in his operative mortality from 40% in 1877 to 14 % in 1884 to 2.4 % in 1889 and 0.18 % in 1898 [6, 7]. He attributed this in part to antiseptic techniques introduced by Lister in 1867 and anaesthesia [5].

The introduction of anaesthesia in the mid 1800's allowed the first successful thyroidectomy to be performed in St. Petersburg by Nikolai Pirigoff. Haemostatic forceps was another remarkable tool introduced at the same time by Spencer Wells and Jules Pear in 1874 [8].

Thyroid surgery evolved from the use of hot setons to destroy thyroid nodules to ligation of arterial poles and finally to excision of the thyroid gland totally or in part.

Damage to the recurrent laryngeal nerve has always been avoided; Billroth, Kocher, and other investigators avoided the nerve and proposed that the inferior thyroid artery should be isolated and ligated laterally to avoid nerve injury. Kocher also left behind the posterior portion of the internal thyroid capsule to avoid the nerve injury. Nerve injuries however were largely unnoticed until the invention of laryngoscopy by Spanish singer Manuel Garcia in 1851 due to his extreme enthusiasm to see inside his throat while singing. Billroth, Kocher, and Joll tried to avoid the nerve at surgery and Frank Lahey, in 1938, advocated that exposure of the nerve routinely resulted in an injury rate of only 0.3% [8].

The importance of superior laryngeal nerve function was realized after the injury to the nerve during the surgery on the famous singer Amelita Galli-Curci. Arnold Kegel and G. Raphael Dunleavy performed this surgery[3].

Thyroid surgery today uses multiple techniques and technology developed over the span of 200 years so that thyroidectomy can even be considered as an outpatient procedure in selected cases [9].

The Anatomy of the Thyroid Gland

This subject has been extensively discussed in our chapter on thyroid anatomy earlier in this book. We looked at the relevant surgical relations and the landmarks used to identify and preserve the recurrent laryngeal nerve (RLN) and external branch of the superior laryngeal nerves (EBSLN) and the parathyroid glands. Beautiful anatomical illustrations were provided which will assist in understanding the principles involved in safe thyroid surgery.

Diagnostic Investigations and Preoperative Preparation

Prior to thyroid surgery the lesion must be accurately diagnosed and malignant disease accurately staged in order to plan the operation and improve outcomes. The distinction between benign and malignant disease governs the type of procedure done and the following investigation may help with this:

Thyroid Ultrasound: A high frequency (7.5-15mHz) probe is used. The sensitivity of ultrasound in identifying asymptomatic nodules is 67% compared to physical examination (5-8%) [10]. Features suggestive of malignancy include marked hypo echogenicity, loss of the associated halo, mixed cystic and solid components, increased vascularity, irregular margins, micro calcifications, length >width and associated cervical lymphadenopathy. The presence of the "halo" sign (a thin hypoechoic rim surrounding a nodule) is very suggestive of benign pathology [11, 12]. Ultrasound is also useful for guided FNAC of the thyroid mass or lymph nodes.

Fine Needle Aspiration for Cytology (FNAC): FNAC differentiates between benign and malignant disease, helps select patients for surgery and governs type of operation done. It can be done under ultrasound guidance for non-palpable nodules, cystic nodules and posterior nodules [13]. Also FNA of suspicious lymph nodes can determine if lymph node dissection should be performed intra operatively [13, 14].

Papillary, medullary, anaplastic carcinoma as well as lymphoma can be reliably diagnosed by FNAC. Follicular or Hurthle cell neoplasms cannot be deemed malignant on FNAC and requires histologic proof of capsular invasion. Papillary cystic nodules that repeatedly yield non-diagnostic aspirates should be considered for surgery as well as solid solitary lesions of indeterminate FNAC. Generally lesions less than 1cm are not investigated with FNAC unless there is a strong suspicion of cancer based on the history, physical findings or ultrasound.

Molecular Diagnostic Testing can be done on indeterminate FNA specimens to identify true carcinomas. These include BRAF, RAS, RET/PTC, Pax8-PPAR gamma, or galectin-3 [13].

Thyroid Scintigraphy (Radio Isotopes or Technetium-99): Although not always necessary this test can be used determine the functional status of a nodule. Non-functioning (cold) and indeterminate nodules should be assessed by FNA. Autonomous (hot/hyper functioning nodules) do not routinely need FNA. The cold nodule is malignant in 15-20% of cases and hot nodules can have malignancy in up to 9% of cases [15]. Technetium can be used to determine function due to its short half-life and it is not organified by the thyroid gland. Radioactive iodine I^{123} and I^{131} are both used for scanning and are organified by the thyroid gland. Both have a longer half life than technetium. I^{123} is used due to its shorter half-life and lower radiation dose. I^{131} can be used to perform the same function but in higher does and is used to ablate residual thyroid tissue left after surgical intervention or for distant metastases.

Computed Tomography (CT) or Magnetic resonance imaging (MRI) can be used to preoperatively stage malignant disease (detect involved lymph nodes, muscle invasion and distant metastases). There should be a 2 month delay between CT with iodine and future radioiodine therapy as contrast may block iodine uptake by thyroid gland and limit the effectiveness of radioiodine therapy[11]. If retrosternal extension is suspected clinically, a CT scan with contrast must be done preoperatively. Imaging is also important to assess vascular invasion by tumours, relationship to the great vessels and the location of the lesion in the mediastinum.

Specific Work up for Medullary Carcinoma

Carcinoembryonic antigen (CEA) and Calcitonin should be measured preoperatively to use as a baseline for comparison after surgery [11, 16].

A patient with medullary thyroid carcinoma should be investigated for Multiple Endocrine Neoplasia Type 2 (MEN2) syndrome. Serum calcium should be done to screen for hyperparathyroidism. The diagnosis of pheochromocytoma can be established by measuring plasma metanephrine levels or through measuring metanephrine in the supine position or catecholamine levels in a 24-hour urine collection [17]. If pheochromocytoma is found it should be removed prior to thyroidectomy [18]. All patients with Medullary thyroid cancer should be offered germ line RET analysis even those who appear to have sporadic mutations [16]. If the patient is positive for the RET proto-oncogene then family members should be screened.

Work up Specific to the Operation

Thyroid surgery may result in numerous intraoperative and postoperative complications. However if a patient is optimized thoroughly prior to surgery some of these complications can be avoided.

Blood Tests	Complete Blood count Group & Cross Match Renal function Liver function Thyroid Function Tests (Serum TSH, Serum free T4, Total T3) Serum Calcium	Should have optimal haemoglobin since intra-operative blood loss may be significant. Patient should be euthyroid at surgery to minimize risk of thyroid storm (see below) Screen for hyperparathyroidism
Evaluate cardiac risk	Functional status Pulse: rhythm and rate Blood pressure. ECG Echocardiogram	Thyroid hormone is positively inotropic, increases stroke volume, cardiac output and left ventricular ejection fraction predisposing to high output cardiac failure, arrhythmias, tachycardia, systolic hypertension and angina
Pulmonary and airway assessment	Chest X Ray Respiratory Flow loops studies	Tracheal deviation, mediastinal extension and pulmonary metastases. Extra thoracic compression of the trachea by a goiter results in flattening of intra thoracic and extra thoracic loops
Pre operative laryngoscopy	To evaluate vocal cords and document adequate function	Important for baseline documentation [19].

Pharmacological Therapy

Hyperthyroidism should be controlled before surgery to minimize adverse cardiovascular outcomes and prevent precipitation of thyroid storm.

The use of the following drugs can render the patient euthyroid prior to surgery:

- Beta blockers (e.g. Atenolol) for control of adrenergic symptoms [20, 21].
- Thionamides: Carbimazole (active metabolite is methimazole) is usually started in patients with biochemical evidence of hyperthyroidism. Propylthiouracil should never be used first line, because of the risk of severe liver injury, except in the following circumstances: the first trimester of pregnancy, for people with minor reactions to carbimazole who refuse treatment with radioactive iodine or surgery and in the treatment of thyroid storm (since it inhibits T4 conversion to the more potent T3) [21].
- Iodine decreases the synthesis of thyroid hormone and decreases the release of thyroid hormone from the gland. In thyrotoxic patients Saturated Solution of potassium Iodine (SSKI) or Lugol's Iodine can be used as an adjunct to antithyroid drugs 10-14 days before surgery to reduce vascularity of the gland and reduce intraoperative blood loss. Thyroid hormone production must first be blocked with thionamides before starting iodine to prevent an iodine-induced thyrotoxicosis. Iodine should not be used in conditions with autonomous thyroid synthesis (e.g. toxic adenoma and toxic multinodular goiter) as they may lead to thyrotoxicosis by the Jod-Basedow phenomenon [20].

General Measures

Prophylaxis of Post Operative Nausea and Vomiting

There is a relatively high incidence of postoperative nausea and vomiting (PONV) with thyroidectomies. Serotonin antagonists, corticosteroids and dopamine antagonists can be used independently or in combination to decrease PONV [22, 23].

Deep Venous Thromboembolism Prophylaxis

Given the high risk of bleeding with thyroidectomies and low risk of deep vein thrombosis (DVT), if no risk factors for DVT are present no routine pharmacological prophylaxis is indicated. Ambulation should be encouraged before surgery and mechanical methods (graduated compression stockings and pneumatic calf compression devices) can be employed [14].

Nursing Post-Operatively

Patients should be nursed in close proximity of the staff in event of major post op bleeding which will cause acute respiratory compromise. Also they should be nursed in a 30-45 degree head elevation. A thyroid tray and crash cart should be close to bedside in the event the incision needs to be opened urgently for bleeding.

Calcium and/or PTH monitoring should be done for patients with symptoms of hypocalcemia or routinely if the dissection of parathyroids was difficult or parathyroids not clearly visualized.

Indications for Thyroid Surgery

Thyroid surgery encompasses a variety of procedures listed below:

- *Hemi-thyroidectomy*: complete removal of one lobe and isthmus
- *Sub-Total-Lobectomy:* Total lobectomy but leaving behind a small amount of thyroid tissue in an effort to protect the recurrent laryngeal nerves
- *Sub-total Thyroidectomy*: Both lobes are removed except for a small amount of thyroid tissue (on one or both sides) in the vicinity of the recurrent laryngeal nerve
- *Total Thyroidectomy*: the removal of both lobes, isthmus and pyramidal lobe
- *Isthmusectomy:* removal of the isthmus
- *Central Lymph Node Dissection*: the removal of the central compartment nodes in event that one is operating for papillary or medullary carcinoma

Table 1. Demonstrating the surgical procedure for various thyroid diseases [11, 13, 18, 20, 21, 24-27]

Disease	Recommended Procedure	Notes
Graves Disease	Total thyroidectomy or sub-total thyroidectomy is equally effective as anti-thyroid medications and radioactive iodine therapy in treating Graves Disease	Consider surgery in patients with 1) Symptoms refractory to thyroid medications and radio-iodine therapy or severe reactions to medical therapy 2) Co-existing pathology (parathyroid disease, thyroid nodule or severe ophthalmopathy) 3) Large goitres with compressive symptoms e.g. dysphagia, dyspnea, hoarseness of voice, inspiratory stridor, pain 4) Symptomatic pregnant patients who are allergic to or experience serious side effects (e.g. agranulocytosis) on thionamides. Surgery in the second trimester may reduce fetal and maternal risks.
Reidel's Thyroiditis	Isthmusectomy	To prevent tracheal compression
Multinodular Non Toxic Goitre	Total or near-total thyroidectomy	Multinodular Non Toxic Goitre
Toxic adenoma	Ipsilateral lobectomy or Isthmusectomy (if adenoma is located in the isthmus)	Consider surgery over radioiodine therapy in 1) Patients with large obstructive goitres 2) Patients who need rapid correction of hyperthyroidism 3) Coexisting malignancy or parathyroid disease 4) Women planning a pregnancy 5) Children
Toxic adenoma and non functioning nodule in other lobe	Total thyroidectomy	
Multinodular Toxic Goitre	Total or sub-total thyroidectomy	
Thyroid Nodules: 1) If repeat FNA shows atypical features or mixed macro- and microfollicular cells 2) follicular neoplasm is suspected or Hurtle cells on FNAC 3) suspicion of malignancy but no definitive diagnosis can be given	Diagnostic Hemi-thyroidectomy with completion thyroidectomy if surgical histology shows follicular thyroid cancer	If scintigraphy or molecular testing is available, may do these before deciding on surgical option.

Table 1. (Continued)

Disease	Recommended Procedure	Notes
Papillary or follicular cancer	Unilateral lobectomy and isthmusectomy (optional but Total Thyroidectomy standard)	Low risk patients, single nodule, <4cm, with no evidence of extra thyroid extension, confined to one lobe or gland, no lymph nodes involved High risk patients, >4cm Presence of multiple tumour nodules, extra thyroid extension or metastases Previously exposed to radioiodine of head and neck If there is no lymph node involvement consider prophylactic central dissection in large tumours (>4cm) If there is confirmed lymph node involvement therapeutic lymph node dissection is indicated
Medullary carcinoma	Total thyroidectomy with central neck node dissection	Consider prophylactic lateral neck dissection if extensive lymph node metastases in central neck or if pre op imaging shows lymph node involvement in the lateral compartment
Multiple Endocrine Neoplasia Type 2 (MEN 2)	Prophylactic thyroidectomy	Timing of surgery is based upon the specific DNA mutation in RET proto-oncogene. Patient stratified into risk group based on codons affected. Highest risk: operate in 1st year of life High risk: 2-4 years Intermediate: before 6 years Low risk: by 10 years or if there is an abnormal calcitonin stimulation test (after provocation with calcium or pentagastrin)
Anaplastic tumours	Total thyroidectomy with post op external beam radiation if no infiltration and extension into surrounding tissue but rarely present at a stage amenable to surgery	In the majority of cases the surgeon's role is primarily to biopsy to diagnose or to secure an airway.
Thyroid Lymphoma	Thyroidectomy of little or no value	Only role of surgeon is diagnostic biopsy

One may embark on thyroid surgery for various benign and malignant conditions which will be discussed below (Table 1). Particularly for benign disease other therapeutic options (radioactive iodine therapy or anti thyroid medications) are available and the treatment should be based on patient factors after review with an endocrinologist and discussion with the patient.

Thyroidectomy Surgical Techniques

Basics

The patient should be supine on the operating table with a sandbag placed at the back between the shoulder blades so the shoulders would droop laterally; a head ring is put behind the extended neck to stabilise the head. The chin should be straight and the shoulders symmetrical. The head of the bed is then elevated 15-20° to decrease venous pressure in the neck. It is preferable for the surgeon to operate with loupe magnification (2.5 – 3.5x) and coaxial head lighting.

Collar Incision

This was first described by the renowned Nobel Prize winning thyroid surgeon, Theodore Kocher. It is a curved, transverse neck incision, 2.0 – 3.0 cm above the sternal notch. Ideally, it should be marked preoperatively, before the neck is extended on the operating table. When the neck is extended, the skin is drawn cranially and a low neck incision could actually be on or below the sternal notch.

These latter incisions often heal with an unsightly scar; it is better to err on the side of placing the incision more cephalad rather than caudad. Another advantage of marking the skin pre-op is that skin creases are less evident when the neck is extended at surgery. Skin marking pre-op also ensures symmetry since in asymmetrical thyroid enlargement it is possible to inadvertently carry the incision further to one side than the other.

Having marked the skin, it should be properly stretched to ensure that the incision is vertical to the skin with no skewing of the knife. The cut should be carried down to the deep cervical fascia ensuring that the platysma is incised throughout the length of the incision and that the anterior jugular veins are preserved.

While meticulous haemostasis is essential, the authors prefer diathermy coagulation over the use of infiltration of an adrenaline solution as the latter produces more bulky and turgid flaps than the softer, pliable flaps.

Raising Flaps

The flaps must be raised deep to platysma. If this is done superficial to platysma, flap ischaemia and necrosis may occur. Even if healing is achieved, fibrosis between the skin and platysma produces unsightly tethering each time the platysma contracts. It must be noted that the platysma is often deficient in the midline and less evident in the obese patient with the short thick neck.

In these cases, one must ensure that the incision goes right down to the deep cervical fascia before lifting the flap. It is easier to find the correct plane laterally than in the midline.

A tissue forceps is placed on each side of the midline of the upper flap, engaging the platysma and subcutaneous fat. Upward traction on these by the assistant, combined with downward pressure by the surgeon's non-cutting hand help to define a relatively avascular plane between the deep fascia and subcutaneous fat. This plane must be developed cephalad up to the thyroid prominence. By a similar technique the inferior flap is raised down to the sternal notch. Care must be taken to avoid injury to the anterior jugular veins and their branches as they lie adherent to the deep cervical fascia (Figure 2). If injured, haemostasis should be secured by suturing rather than diathermy. The flaps are then held apart by a thyroid retractor (e.g., Joll's).

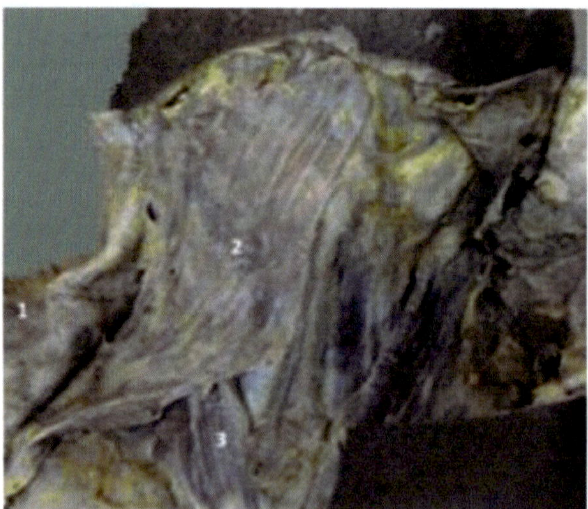

Figure 1. Photograph of the neck of a human cadaver. The skin and subcutaneous tissues (1) have been reflected to reveal the large flat sheet of the platysma muscle (2). Beneath the platysma, the origin of the sternomastoid (3) can be seen on the right.

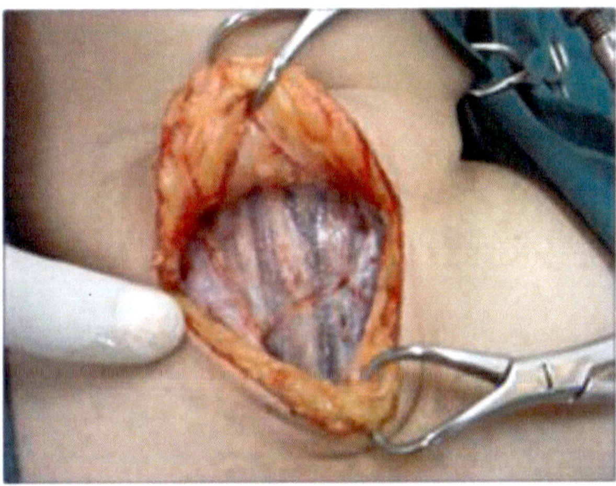

Figure 2. Flaps raised with preservation of the anterior jugular veins.

Exposing the Thyroid

The deep cervical fascia should be incised along the midline. It could be difficult to identify the midline especially in asymmetrical enlargement. It is easier to find the midline by incising the deep fascia near the sternal notch or the thyroid prominence. At both these points the sternothyroid muscle is fixed while the sternohyoid is attached at the lower end.

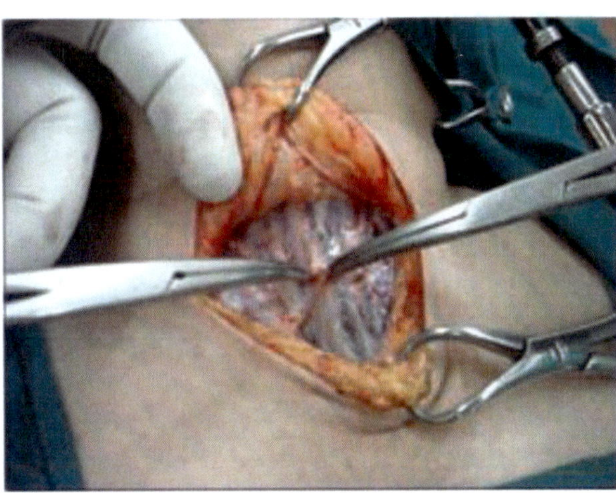

Figure 3. Incision of deep cervical fascia in midline.

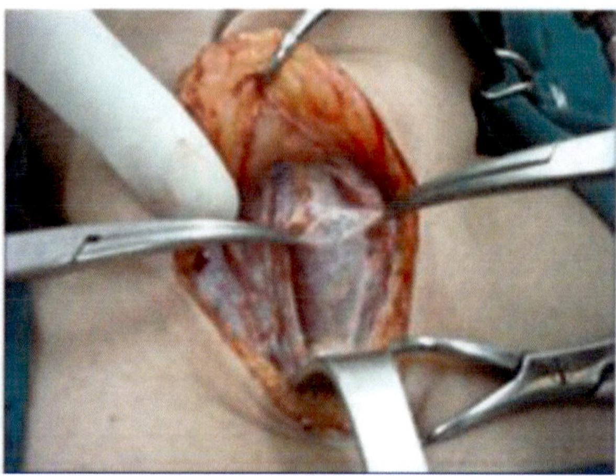

Figure 4. Incision of pretracheal fascia after separation of strap muscles.

The deep cervical fascia is picked up on each side of the midline and lifted with artery forceps (Figure 3). If diathermy coagulation is used to incise this fascia, the contraction of the underlying sternohyoid may assist in identifying the midline. After the fascial incision is carried from the thyroid prominence to the sternal notch, the strap muscles are separated in the midline. When the thyroid isthmus is approached, the pretracheal fascia should be lifted with artery forceps and incised sharply (Figure 4).

Care should be taken that this layer is opened for the full length of the incision. The surgeon should now stand on the side opposite to the lobe being mobilised. The strap muscles and deep fascia of the side being exposed are grasped by two tissue forceps and lifted. The surgeon depresses the thyroid with one hand while incising the plane between the deep surface of the sternothyroid muscle and the thyroid capsule. This should be done meticulously while coagulating the few small vessels that traverse this plane. When the dissection has extended about 2cm laterally, the tissue forceps are removed and two US Army/Navy retractors used to expose the anterolateral aspect of the thyroid lobe. This dissection should be carried as far cephalad and caudad as possible.

Mobilization of Lobe

Medial traction on the thyroid lobe and lateral retraction of the strap muscles should reveal the middle thyroid vein when it is present (in 60 – 70%

cases). The vein should be ligated and divided. In many cases, however, when the lobe is quite large, the space between the lobe and the strap muscles may be too narrow to allow easy access to the vein. In such cases, the whole lobe above and below the middle thyroid vein is mobilized with finger dissection. Then the finger is used to tear the vein off the thyroid lobe as it is delivered into the wound; the lateral aspect of the wound is packed with two small gauze swabs while a swab is kept on the thyroid with the hand drawing the lobe medially. (We found it quite unnecessary to divide the strap muscles in 99% of our last 500 cases.) At this stage, it is possible to peel off the areolar tissue posteromedially to reveal the parathyroids, inferior thyroid artery and recurrent laryngeal nerve (Figure 5).

While the retractors hold the two gauze swabs laterally, the inferior thyroid veins are ligated and divided.

The lower pole is lifted and capsular dissection proceeds cephalad using bipolar cautery; dissection should be maintained closely against the thyroid capsule at all times. When the level of the isthmus is reached this is lifted off the trachea by blunt dissection and the isthmus divided using diathermy coagulation. (Figure 6)

At the superior border of the isthmus, there is an arterial arcade extending from the medial border of each superior pole (across the isthmus); this may need suture ligation.

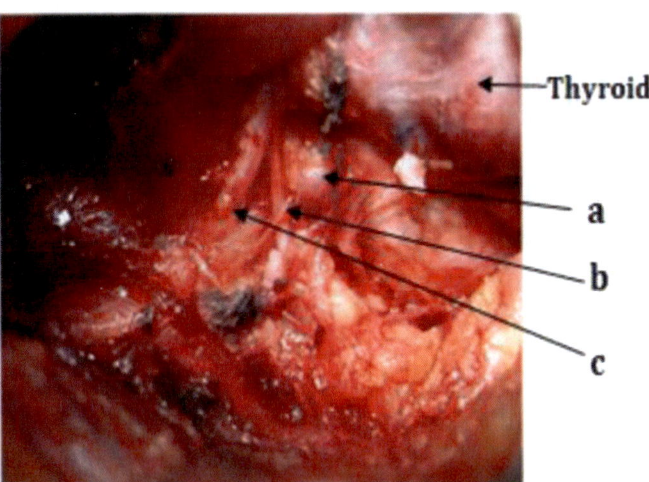

Figure 5. Medical mobilization of the lobe reveals parathyroid (a), RLN (b) and inferior thyroid artery (c).

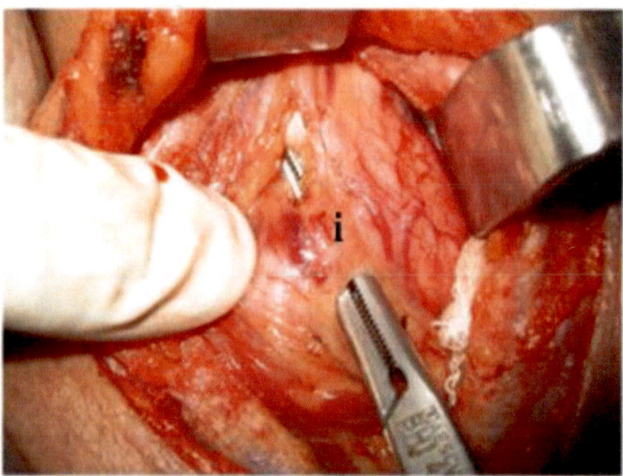

Figure 6. Artery forceps separating isthmus (i) from trachea, facilitating division.

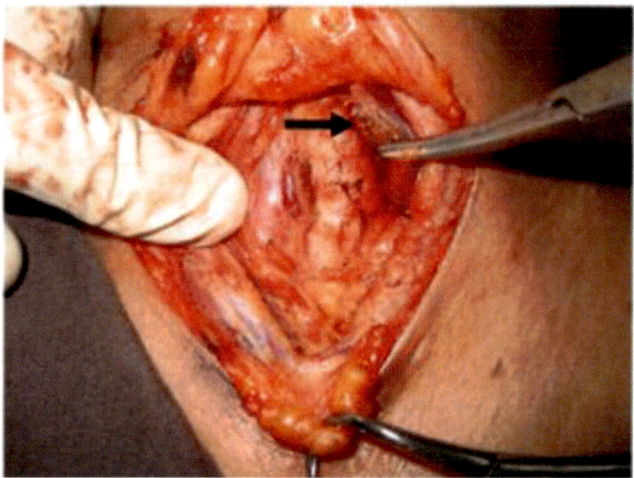

Figure 7. Mobilization of the lobe of the trachea reveals the medial border of the ligament of Berry (arrow).

As the isthmus and lower lobe are lifted off the trachea, the ligament of Berry (LB) is encountered (Figure 7).

This is a firm band of connective tissue that runs from the inner, deep surface of the lateral lobe to the cricoid cartilage. It may also have fibres attaching it to the inferior margin of the thyroid cartilage [28]. This LB must be divided carefully, from medial to lateral, using fine bipolar diathermy forceps.

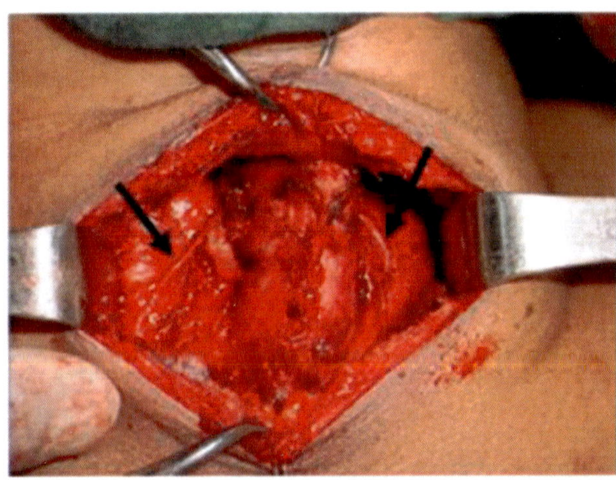

Figure 8. Both RLN's are quite lateral to the tracheo-oesophageal groove in this patient (arrows).

When the lateral portion of the ligament is reached the gland is lifted and the remaining portion is divided from lateral to medial, the dissection being carried out against the deep surface of the gland itself. This is the point where the recurrent laryngeal nerve (RLN) is most vulnerable as it runs immediately posterolateral to the LB and extends about 2mm cephalad before disappearing beneath the inferior constrictor. Although the RLN usually runs in the tracheo-oesophageal groove, it can be quite lateral (Figure 8).

With this lateral edge of the LB taut, under tension, as the thyroid is lifted, it 'snaps open' when divided. If capsular dissection is maintained throughout using bipolar cautery against the gland, it is not necessary to identify the RLN although when the lateral aspect of LB is being divided, the nerve comes into view. In over 50% of cases, a lateral extension of the thyroid lobe, the tubercle of Zuckerkandl may be encountered at this point.

Dissection of this tubercle must be carefully done as the RLN runs immediately deep to it; rarely, the nerve is superficial to it. The thyroid lobe is now fully mobilised by developing the avascular plane of loose areolar tissue between the upper lobe and the cricothyroid muscle. The upper pole is drawn down and the superior pole vessels are peeled free of all areolar tissue with peanut/finger dissection. They are now well visualised and easily ligated and divided (Figure 10).

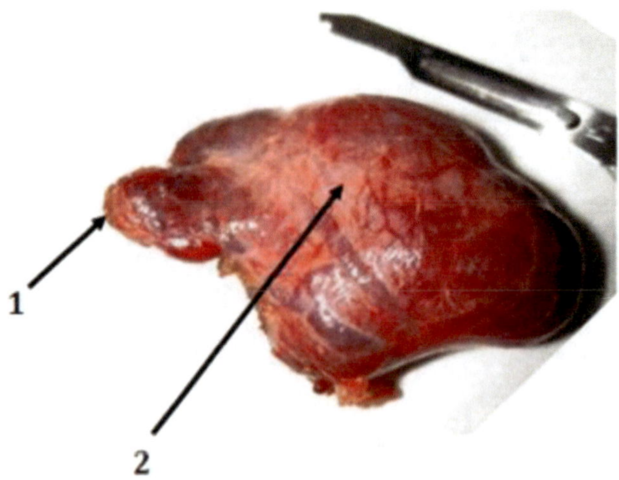

Figure 9. An excised specimen after right hemithyroidectomy. The thyroid gland has been transected at the isthmus. A large Tubercle of Zuckerkandl (1) can be seen at the posterolateral part of the right lateral lobe (2).

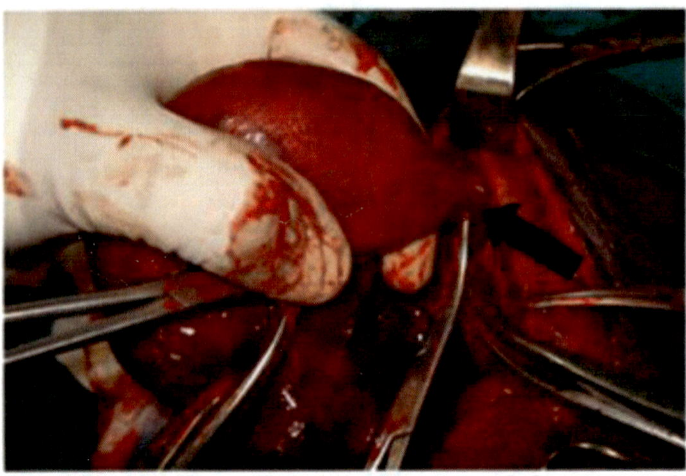

Figure 10. Excellent exposure of the superior thyroid pedicle (arrow) by downward traction of the completely mobilized lobe.

Using this technique of 'retrograde thyroidectomy', the entire lobe and superior thyroid vessels are drawn so far inferiorly that the risk of damage to the external branch of the superior laryngeal nerve (EBSLN) is almost eliminated since the nerve is fixed by its entry into the cricothyroid muscle; the EBSLN can be identified in most cases [29].

For a total thyroidectomy, the same procedure is repeated, with the surgeon moving to the opposite side of the table. In these cases, it is easier to do the larger lobe first.

Subtotal Lobectomy

For subtotal lobectomy, the mobilisation is the same (as above) up to the division of the middle thyroid vein. The lobe is then drawn medially and by blunt (peanut or finger) dissection the lobe is mobilised off the carotid sheath and oesophagus, keeping the plane very close to the thyroid capsule. The inferior thyroid veins are thus divided thus freeing the lower pole.

The upper pole is now mobilised by placing two US Army/Navy retractors laterally and bluntly (using finger/peanut) dissection the lateral and posterior surfaces of the lobe. After thorough lateral and posterior mobilisation, the lower retractor is moved to the midline superiorly so that both sides of the upper pole are exposed. The upper pole is then drawn laterally by the surgeon and the plane between cricothyroid and the upper pole developed by blunt dissection. By this manoeuvre, the upper pole is completely encircled. It must be drawn caudally as far as possible, while gently peeling off all tissue from the superior thyroid pedicle, which is then doubly ligated close to the gland, in continuity, prior to division.

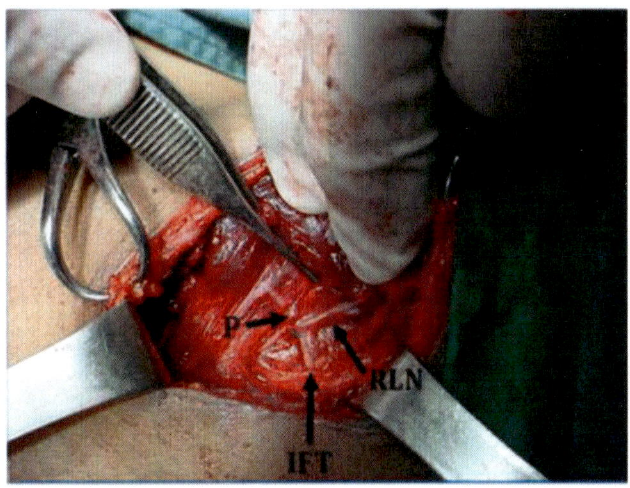

Figure 11. The RLN and parathyroids (P) are preserved if the posteromedial portion of the lobe is not removed. Note: Inferior Thyroid Artery (IFT).

The isthmus is now divided. Thus, the entire lobe apart from its posteromedial attachment is freed. Preservation of this posteromedial portion of the lobe minimises injury to parathyroids and RLN (Figure 11).

Artery forceps are now placed around the lobe at the planned site of resection. These assist with haemostasis but, more importantly, they serve as markers for safe placement of sutures, even if the field is bloody, after transecting the lobe. The thyroid is now resected, constructing a shallow V-wedge if possible. The cut surface is now sutured using a lubricated continuous absorbable suture ensuring adequate bites on both sides of the thyroid tissue and capsule. This ensures good haemostasis. We prefer this technique over the recommendation to suture the cut surface to the trachea.

The wound is closed with continuous suture in 3 layers - deep cervical fascia, platysma and subcuticular, with no drainage [8].

Retrosternal Goitre

If retrosternal extension is suspected clinically, a CT scan with contrast must be done preoperatively. (Figures 12, 13)

This must be studied by the surgeon to ascertain the following:

1. Which lobe(s) extends retrosternally.
2. Depth of extension.
3. Relationship with innominate vein.
4. Any blood supply from within chest.
5. Relationship with trachea, aortic arch and great vessels.

In most retrosternal goitres the lower pole can be delivered by blunt mobilisation with a finger and the thyroidectomy performed with minimal alteration in technique.

While one should always be prepared for thoracotomy, this is particularly relevant when the intra thoracic portion reaches below the aortic arch, is too large to deliver through the thoracic inlet or where malignancy is suspected (and invasion of adjacent structures needs to be considered).

If the retrosternal extension cannot be easily delivered by sweeping the finger around the lower pole, then all suprasternal thyroid tissue must be fully mobilised. This is done by division of the superior pedicle, division of the LB and capsular dissection until the lobe has no attachment on the neck. The thyroid is held with gauze in one hand exercising gentle traction while the

dissecting finger sweeps around the lower pole with great care to ensure that the plane is well defined and the pressure is directed against the thyroid, not on the mediastinal structures. If, in spite of these manoeuvres, the lobe cannot be delivered, the cervical leverage technique (using a US Army/Navy retractor) may be used [30]. If this fails, one may consider using the Marzouk technique or proceed to thoracotomy [31].

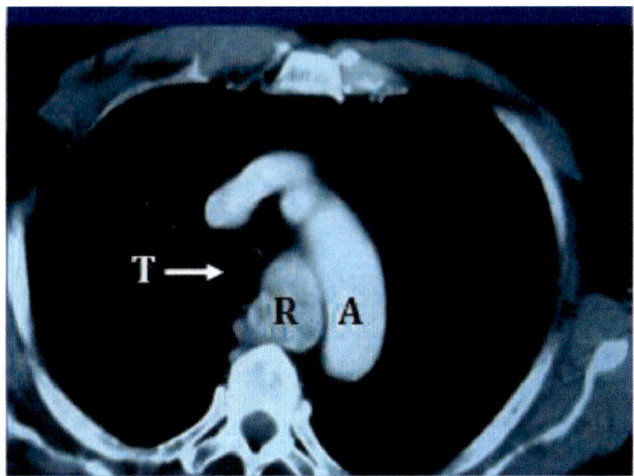

Figure 12. Retrosternal goitre (R) extending between the aortic arch (A) and trachea (T).

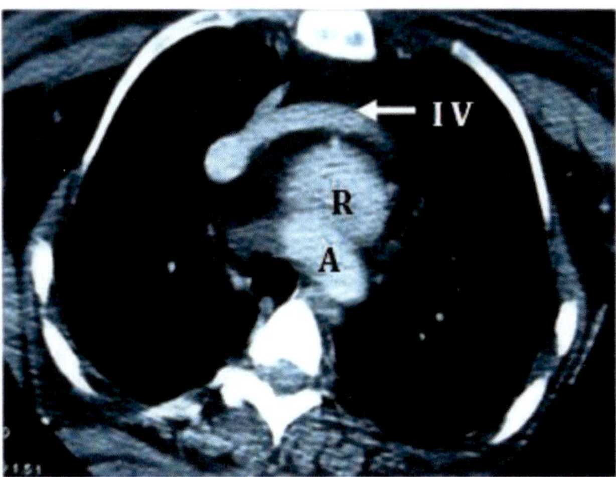

Figure 13. Retrosternal goitre (R) extending between the innominate vein (IV) and aortic arch (A).

Central Node Dissection

Essentially, the central compartment node dissection involves all nodal structures below the hyoid bone, medial to common carotid vessels and superior to the innominate vessels [32, 33]. This is generally segment VI. It is important to identify and protect the recurrent laryngeal nerves inferiorly [32]. Sometimes it may be necessary to remove and re-implant the inferior parathyroids. However this has to be histologically confirmed by frozen section first. The size of the primary tumor guides the use of unilateral or bilateral central dissection with 1cm being the cutoff. A modified radical neck dissection is indicated if there are positive nodes present in segments II-IV [33]. This discussion however is outside the scope of this chapter.

Complications of Thyroidectomy

When Kocher first performed thyroid surgery in 1872 the mortality rate was 75%. At the time the operation was considered so dangerous that it was prohibited by the Academy of Medicine [34].

Fortunately thanks to advances in surgery mortality and morbidity is significantly reduced. However even with experienced surgeons and meticulous care complications still occur. The difficulty of the surgery increases with re-operative thyroidectomy and patients who present late with large infiltrative tumours [35, 36].

Proper preoperative screening, optimisation of patients, sound anatomy, good exposure, and meticulous attention to haemostasis, identification and preservation of the parathyroid glands and laryngeal nerves reduce morbidity and mortality. We will now discuss some of the common complications of thyroidectomy.

Nerve Injury

Identification of the nerves is fundamental to avoid injury [19]. This may be difficult with sub sternal goitre, thyroid cancers, large multinodular goitre and where there are anatomical variations in the nerve's course. Many centres use intraoperative nerve monitoring using electrical stimulation to determine physiological status of the nerve [19, 37]. After identifying and stimulating the nerve the thyroid gland is then removed.

If a recurrent nerve injury becomes apparent intraoperatively, attempts should be made to repair it. Injury of the recurrent laryngeal nerve (RLN) may result in immobile vocal cord, a husky voice, feeble bovine cough and a slightly restricted airway; bilateral RLN injury may present with severe dyspnoea and inspiratory stridor indicating airway obstruction and the patient may require a tracheostomy [24].

The external branch of the superior laryngeal nerve (EBSLN) may be damaged at time of ligation of superior thyroid artery. Injury may be asymptomatic or there may be changes in voice pitch, range and projection.

Transient neuropraxia resolves in weeks to months, while temporary paresis from pressure or traction takes 3 – 6 months to recover. If symptoms persist beyond one year they are likely to be permanent [24].

Tracheal Collapse

This is a very rare complication but can occur when there is loss of elasticity of tracheal cartilage and tracheomalacia from a long standing goiter, with tracheal collapse post-operatively [24]. Treatment involves a tracheostomy.

Hematoma

Post-operative neck hematoma is a surgical emergency [38]. The patient may present 6 to 8 hours post operatively with difficulty breathing and inspiratory stridor due to respiratory obstruction [24]. The hematoma should be evacuated immediately and the patient transferred to the operating room where the neck is explored with an aim to achieve haemostasis.

It should be noted that bilateral cord paralysis, tracheal collapse and hematoma all present with respiratory distress.

Infection

Infection is rare because of good blood supply and perioperative antibiotics are seldom given in immunocompetent patients [24, 39].

Hypocalcaemia Secondary to Hypoparathyroidism (Hungry Bone Syndrome)

Hypoparathyroidism may occur secondary to gland removal or damage to their blood supply, thus attempts should be made to identify and preserve the glands and the vascular pedicles. It is thought that temporary ischemia of the parathyroid gland may result in transient hypocalcemia but permanent hypoparathyroidism also occurs.

Loss of parathyroid hormone encourages rapid remineralisation of bone with precipitous drops in calcium, magnesium and phosphate levels. At end of surgery the specimen should be inspected for parathyroid glands and auto transplantation can be done. Following auto transplantation the patient should be on calcium and vitamin D (alfacalcidol/calcitrol) for 2 to 3 months [24].

Hypocalcaemia may result in tingling in extremities or lips, a positive Trousseau and Chvostek sign, nausea vomiting, thirst, irritability and QT prolongation on electrocardiogram.

Hypocalcaemia can be ascertained by clinical evaluation and serial calcium monitoring post operatively. More recently it has been shown that parathyroid level the morning after surgery was a good predictor for hypocalcaemia [40].

Hypocalcaemic patients should be started on oral calcium and alfacalcidol/calcitrol supplementation based on calcium and parathyroid levels. If calcium levels are very low or refractory to oral supplements intravenous calcium gluconate should be given. A low salt diet may reduce tubular reabsorption of calcium in the kidneys thereby minimising loss in urine[24]. Magnesium and phosphate levels should also be corrected.

Thyroid Storm

Manipulation of the thyroid gland may lead to the release of hormones and precipitate a thyroid crisis. The patient may be distressed, dyspnoeic, tachycardia, hyperexic, with vomiting, diarrhoea, confusion and delirium [18].

Treatment entails intravenous propylthiouracil and propranolol administration under ECG monitoring, the use of super saturated potassium iodine (SSKI) or Lugol's iodine and intravenous hydrocortisone. Supportive measures include intravenous fluids, cooling, oxygen and treatment of cardiac failure [18, 21].

Miscellaneous complications reported include seromas, hypertrophic and keloid scars, Horner's syndrome, chyle fistula and tracheal and oesophageal injury [18, 41, 42].

Advances in Thyroidectomy

Thyroid disease is classically a disease affecting mostly female patients and this has fueled the desire for more cosmetically appropriate approaches [43]. This is of special importance in the dark skinned population where the likelihood of keloid and hypertrophic scarring is increased. Conventional open thyroidectomy has average skinfold incision length of 5-6cm; in minimally invasive open thyroid surgery the average incision length is 3.5 to 4.5cm; compared to endoscopic minimally invasive video assisted thyroid surgery with an incision length less than 2cm [44-47].

In 1997 the first endoscopic approach to thyroid surgery was described by Huscher [48]. In 2000 Miccoli described video assisted techniques using incisions of about 15mm placed 1cm above the sternal notch with CO2 inflation [49]. Since then minimally invasive video assisted thyroid surgery (MIVAT) has been explored by many different studies using a variety of approaches with varying results.

Endoscopic access has been attempted via cervical, axillary and breast approach, with bilateral breast access being favoured as it provides wider access, more range of movement and better cosmetic outcome, as there is no scarring above the neck [40]. Tan et al. reported that the extra-cervical approaches have been associated with longer operating times, increased perioperative morbidity and longer hospital stay. Other centres have found an increase in transient vocal cord palsy and increased transient hypocalcaemia but similar rates in other complications compared to open thyroidectomy [40].

Robotic technology has also been applied to thyroid surgery using a gasless unilateral axillo-breast or axillary approach with a Da Vinci robotic system (described by Kang et al) [50]. Robotic surgery has proven itself to be a reasonable and safe alternative to open and endoscopic procedure however there is increased cost.

One key factor to consider when evaluating the benefit of endoscopic or robotic surgery is the competency of the surgeon with the equipment. The learning curve for performing these procedures is significantly greater than open thyroidectomy and operating time can be significantly increased when performed by inexperienced surgeons, however they may have better cosmesis, less postoperative pain, and reduced hospital stay [44, 47].

In conclusion as with most things in medicine each case must be evaluated holistically. With the right patient selection and in competent hands endoscopic and robotic technology are reasonable minimally invasive options for thyroid surgery and can provide cosmetically favourable results.

References

[1] Contin P, Goossen K, Grummich K, et al. ENERgized vessel sealing systems versus CONventional hemostasis techniques in thyroid surgery--the ENERCON systematic review and network meta-analysis. *Langenbeck's archives of surgery / Deutsche Gesellschaft fur Chirurgie.* Dec 2013; 398(8):1039-1056.

[2] Cheng LHH, Hutchison IL. Thyroid surgery. *The British journal of oral & maxillofacial surgery.* 2012; 50(7):585-591.

[3] Dorairajan N, Pradeep PV. Vignette Thyroid Surgery: A Glimpse Into its History. *International Surgery.* 2013/02/01 2013; 98(1):70-75.

[4] Shuja A. History of Thryoid Surgery. *The Professional Medical Journal* June 2008 2008; 15(02):295-297.

[5] Dubhashi SP, Subnis BM, Sindwani RD. Theodor e. Kocher. *The Indian journal of surgery.* Oct 2013; 75(5):383-384.

[6] Halsted W. *The Operative Story of Goitre*1920.

[7] Gemsenjäger E. Milestones in European Thyroidology: Theodor Kocher (1841-1917) *European Thyroid Association.*

[8] Daniel O, Robert U. Surgery of the Thyroid and Parathyroid Glands. In: Daniel O, Robert U, eds: Springer Berlin Heidelberg; 2007.

[9] Hessman C, Fields J, Schuman E. Outpatient thyroidectomy: is it a safe and reasonable option? *The American Journal of Surgery.* 5// 2011; 201(5): 565-569.

[10] Tan GH, Gharib H. Thyroid incidentalomas: management approaches to nonpalpable nodules discovered incidentally on thyroid imaging. *Annals of internal medicine.* Feb 1 1997; 126(3):226-231.

[11] Perros P. Guidelines for the Management of Thyroid cancer (Third Edition). *British Thyroid Association.* 2014.

[12] Fish SA, Langer JE, Mandel SJ. Sonographic imaging of thyroid nodules and cervical lymph nodes. *Endocrinology and metabolism clinics of North America.* Jun 2008; 37(2):401-417, ix.

[13] American Thyroid Association Guidelines Taskforce on Thyroid N, Differentiated Thyroid C, Cooper DS, et al. Revised American Thyroid Association management guidelines for patients with thyroid nodules and differentiated thyroid cancer. *Thyroid : official journal of the American Thyroid Association.* Nov 2009; 19(11):1167-1214.

[14] Perros P, Thyroid Cancer Guidelines Update G. Introduction to the updated guidelines on the management of thyroid cancer. *Clinical medicine.* Aug 2007; 7(4):321-322.

[15] Townsend C, Beauchamp R, Evers B. The biological Basis of Modern Surgical Practice 19th Ed *Sabiston Textbook of Surgery Elsevier* 2012.

[16] American Thyroid Association Guidelines Task F, Kloos RT, Eng C, et al. Medullary thyroid cancer: management guidelines of the American Thyroid Association. *Thyroid : official journal of the American Thyroid Association.* Jun 2009; 19(6):565-612.

[17] Chen H, Sippel RS, O'Dorisio MS, Vinik AI, Lloyd RV, Pacak K. The North American Neuroendocrine Tumor Society consensus guideline for the diagnosis and management of neuroendocrine tumors: pheochromocytoma, paraganglioma, and medullary thyroid cancer. *Pancreas.* Aug 2010; 39(6):775-783.

[18] Lennard T. *Endocrine Surgery* 4th ed: Elsevier; 2009.

[19] Chandrasekhar SS, Randolph GW, Seidman MD, et al. Clinical practice guideline: improving voice outcomes after thyroid surgery. *Otolaryngology--head and neck surgery : official journal of American Academy of Otolaryngology-Head and Neck Surgery.* Jun 2013; 148(6 Suppl):S1-37.

[20] Langley RW, Burch HB. Perioperative management of the thyrotoxic patient. *Endocrinology and metabolism clinics of North America.* Jun 2003; 32(2):519-534.

[21] Bahn RS, Burch HB, Cooper DS, et al. Hyperthyroidism and other causes of thyrotoxicosis: management guidelines of the American Thyroid Association and American Association of Clinical Endocrinologists. *Endocrine practice : official journal of the American College of Endocrinology and the American Association of Clinical Endocrinologists.* May-Jun 2011; 17(3):456-520.

[22] Danner K, Becker HG, Best B, Madler C. [Prophylaxis of nausea and vomiting after thyroid surgery: comparison of oral and intravenous dolasetron with intravenous droperidol and placebo]. *Anasthesiologie, Intensivmedizin, Notfallmedizin, Schmerztherapie : AINS.* Jul 2001; 36(7): 425-430.

[23] Zhou H, Xu H, Zhang J, Wang W, Wang Y, Hu Z. Combination of dexamethasone and tropisetron before thyroidectomy to alleviate postoperative nausea, vomiting, and pain: randomized controlled trial. *World journal of surgery*. Jun 2012; 36(6):1217-1224.

[24] Shaheen O. *Thyroid Surgery*: The Parthenon Publishing Group 2003.

[25] Douglas S, Sonia L. Surgery in the Treatment of hyperthyroidism: Indications, preoperative preparation, and post operative followup *UpToDate*. 2014.

[26] Cornelis J. Approach to Therapy in Multiple Endocrine Neeoplasia Type 2. *UpToDate*. 2012.

[27] Nixon IJ, Ganly I, Shah JP. Thyroid cancer: surgery for the primary tumor. *Oral oncology*. Jul 2013; 49(7):654-658.

[28] Yalçın B, Ozan H. Detailed Investigation of the Relationship Between the Inferior Laryngeal Nerve Including Laryngeal Branches and Ligament of Berry. *Journal of the American College of Surgeons. 2//* 2006; 202(2):291-296.

[29] Friedman M, LoSavio P, Ibrahim H. SUperior laryngeal nerve identification and preservation in thyroidectomy. *Archives of Otolaryngology–Head & Neck Surgery*. 2002; 128(3):296-303.

[30] Naraynsingh V, Ramarine I, Cawich SO, Maharaj R, Dan D. Cervical leverage: A new procedure to deliver deep retrosternal goitres without thoracotomy. *International Journal of Surgery Case Reports. //* 2013; 4(11):992-996.

[31] Rathinam S, Davies B, Khalil-Marzouk JF. Marzouk's Procedure: A Novel Combined Cervical and Anterior Mediastinotomy Technique to Avoid Median Sternotomy for Difficult Retrosternal Thyroidectomy. *The Annals of Thoracic Surgery*. 8// 2006; 82(2):759-760.

[32] Hughes DT, Doherty GM. Central neck dissection for papillary thyroid cancer. *Cancer control : journal of the Moffitt Cancer Center*. Apr 2011; 18(2):83-88.

[33] American Thyroid Association Surgery Working G, American Association of Endocrine S, American Academy of O-H, et al. Consensus statement on the terminology and classification of central neck dissection for thyroid cancer. *Thyroid : official journal of the American Thyroid Association*. Nov 2009; 19(11):1153-1158.

[34] Chiesa F. The 100 years Anniversary of the Nobel Prize Award winner Emil Theodor Kocher, a brilliant far-sighted surgeon. *Acta otorhinolaryngologica Italica : organo ufficiale della Societa italiana di otorinolaringologia e chirurgia cervico-facciale*. Dec 2009; 29(6):289.

[35] Gopalakrishna Iyer N, Shaha AR. Reoperative Thyroid Surgery. *Thyroid Surgery*: John Wiley & Sons, Ltd; 2012:105-110.

[36] Lefevre JH, Tresallet C, Leenhardt L, Jublanc C, Chigot JP, Menegaux F. Reoperative surgery for thyroid disease. *Langenbeck's archives of surgery / Deutsche Gesellschaft fur Chirurgie.* Nov 2007; 392(6):685-691.

[37] NICE. Intraopertive Nerve Monitoring During Thyroid Surgery. *National Institute for Health and Clinical Excellence.* March 2008 2008.

[38] Williams RT, Angelos P. Postoperative Bleeding. *Thyroid Surgery*: John Wiley & Sons, Ltd; 2012:199-207.

[39] Avenia N, Sanguinetti A, Cirocchi R, et al. Antibiotic prophylaxis in thyroid surgery: a preliminary multicentric Italian experience. *Annals of surgical innovation and research.* 2009; 3:10.

[40] Dhepnorrarat RC, Witterick IJ. New technologies in thyroid cancer surgery. *Oral oncology.* Jul 2013; 49(7):659-664.

[41] Alon EE, Urken ML. Management and Prevention of Laryngotracheal and Oesophageal Injuries in Thyroid Surgery. *Thyroid Surgery*: John Wiley & Sons, Ltd; 2012:151-160.

[42] Kus LH, Freeman JL. The Rare Ones: Horner's Syndrome, Complications from Surgical Positioning and Post-Sternotomy Complications. *Thyroid Surgery*: John Wiley & Sons, Ltd; 2012:237-248.

[43] Giannopoulos G, Kang SW, Jeong JJ, Nam KH, Chung WY. Robotic thyroidectomy for benign thyroid diseases: a stepwise strategy to the adoption of robotic thyroidectomy (gasless, transaxillary approach). *Surgical laparoscopy, endoscopy & percutaneous techniques.* Jun 2013; 23(3):312-315.

[44] Timon C, Rafferty M. Minimally invasive video-assisted thyroidectomy (MIVAT): technique, advantages, and disadvantages. *Operative Techniques in Otolaryngology-Head and Neck Surgery.* 3// 2008; 19(1): 8-14.

[45] Rafferty M, Timon C. Minimal incision thyroidectomy. *Operative Techniques in Otolaryngology-Head and Neck Surgery.* 3// 2008; 19(1): 2-7.

[46] Brunaud L, Zarnegar R, Wada N, Ituarte P, Clark OH, Duh QY. Incision length for standard thyroidectomy and parathyroidectomy: when is it minimally invasive? *Archives of surgery (Chicago, Ill. : 1960).* Oct 2003; 138(10):1140-1143.

[47] Miccoli P, Berti P, Raffaelli M, Materazzi G, Baldacci S, Rossi G. Comparison between minimally invasive video-assisted thyroidectomy and conventional thyroidectomy: A prospective randomized study. *Surgery.* 12// 2001; 130(6):1039-1043.

[48] Hüscher CS, Chiodini S, Napolitano C, Recher A. Endoscopic right thyroid lobectomy. *Surgical endoscopy.* 08/ 1997; 11(8):877.

[49] Miccoli P, Berti P, Bendinelli C, Conte M, Fasolini F, Martino E. Minimally invasive video-assisted surgery of the thyroid: a preliminary report. *Langenbeck's Arch. Surg.* 2000/07/01 2000; 385(4):261-264.

[50] Kang S-W, Lee SC, Lee SH, et al. Robotic thyroid surgery using a gasless, transaxillary approach and the da Vinci S system: The operative outcomes of 338 consecutive patients. *Surgery.* 12// 2009; 146(6):1048-1055.

In: Thyroidectomy
Editor: Kimberly Rodolfo
ISBN: 978-1-63321-440-8

Chapter 6

Surgical Anatomy of the Thyroid and Parathyroid Glands: A Pictorial Review with Clinical Correlates

Shamir O. Cawich*[1]*, Michael T. Gardner*[2]*,
***Dilip Dan*[1]*, Vijay Naraynsingh*[1] *and Ramanand Shetty*[2]**
[1]Department of Clinical Surgical Sciences, Faculty of Medical Sciences, University of the West Indies, St Augustine Campus, St Augustine, Trinidad and Tobago, West Indies
[2]Department of Basic Medical Sciences, Faculty of Medical Sciences, University of the West Indies, Mona Campus, Mona, Kingston, Jamaica, West Indies

Abstract

The first reports of thyroid surgery can be traced back to the 12th century, when only crude operative methods and rudimentary anaesthetic techniques were available. Theodor Kocher revolutionized the thyroid-dectomy technique in 1877 by introducing meticulous dissection and better antisepsis techniques.

In the 1890's William Halsted, Charles Mayo and George Crile popularized Kocher's techniques in the United States.

Operative morbidity reduced further with technical refinements made by Thomas Dunhill who introduced capsular dissection in 1912 and Frank Lahey who popularized nerve preservation in 1938.

By the late 20th century there were significant advances in pharmacology, anaesthetic techniques and antisepsis. Coupled with refined operative techniques and meticulous dissection, thyroidectomy is now a safe operation with complication rates less than 1%.

To ensure good outcomes, surgeons performing thyroidectomy must be acutely familiar with the anatomy, and common varations of the thyroid gland. In this chapter we review the gross anatomy of the gland, with special emphasis on the surgical importance of the structures encountered during a thyroidectomy. We discuss the anatomic basis of the operative techniques and the common variations that may be encountered when performing a thyroidectomy.

Introduction

The first reports of thyroid surgery can be traced back to the 12th century [1]. The associated mortality at that time was unacceptable because only crude operative methods were available and anaesthesia and antisepsis were in their infancy. It was not until 1877 when Theodor Kocher began to perform thyroidectomies in Germany with meticulous dissection techniques that the operative mortality reduced from over 40% [2] to 13% [3].

In the 1890's William Halsted, Charles Mayo and George Crile popularized Kocher's operative techniques in the United States [2].

Operative morbidity reduced further with technical refinements made by Thomas Dunhill who introduced capsular dissection in 1912 [4] and Frank Lahey who emphasized nerve preservation in 1938 [5].

By the mid-20th century there were significant advances in pharmacology, anaesthetic techniques and antisepsis.

Coupled with refined operative techniques and meticulous dissection, thyroidectomy is now considered a safe operation with complication rates less than 1% [6].

To ensure good outcomes, surgeons performing thyroidectomy must be intimately familiar with the anatomy of the thyroid gland.

In this chapter we review the gross anatomy, with special emphasis on the surgical importance of the structures encountered during a thyroidectomy. We discuss the anatomic basis of the operative techniques and the common variations that may be encountered when performing a thyroidectomy.

Surgical Anatomy of the Thyroid Gland

The thyroid gland is located in the neck deep to the platysma (Figure 1). This is a broad sheet of muscle that crosses over the clavicle to cover the antero-lateral neck. Its anterior fibres interlace with the opposite side, finding an attachment to the mandible and the dermis of the lower part of the face. The platymsa covers the sternocleidomastoid (Figure 2) and the strap muscles of the neck: sternothyroid, sternohyoid and omohyoid (Figures 3 and 4).

The thyroid gland lies in the anterior neck deep to these muscles (Figure 5) and the anterior layer of cervical fascia [7]. The strap muscles meet, but do not cross the midline of the neck.

In order to maximize aesthetics after thyroidectomy, surgeons use a transverse collar incision through the skin and platysma. The deep cervical fascia, however, is incised vertically in the midline to avoid bleeding from the strap muscles of the neck that are running parallel in a sagittal plane.

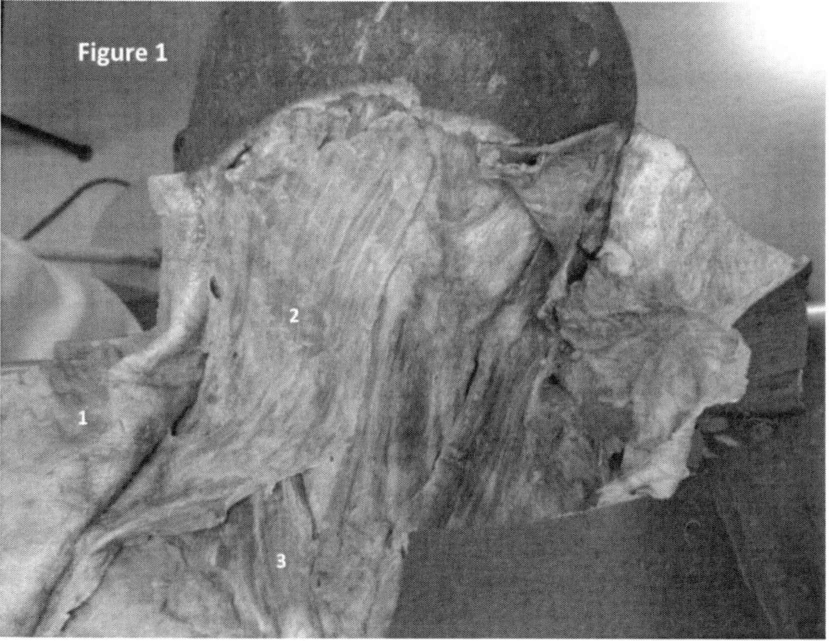

Figure 1. Photograph of the neck of a human cadaver. The skin and subcutaneous tissues (1) have been reflected to reveal the large flat sheet of platysma muscle (2). Beneath the platysma, the origin of sternomastoid muscle (3) can be seen on the right.

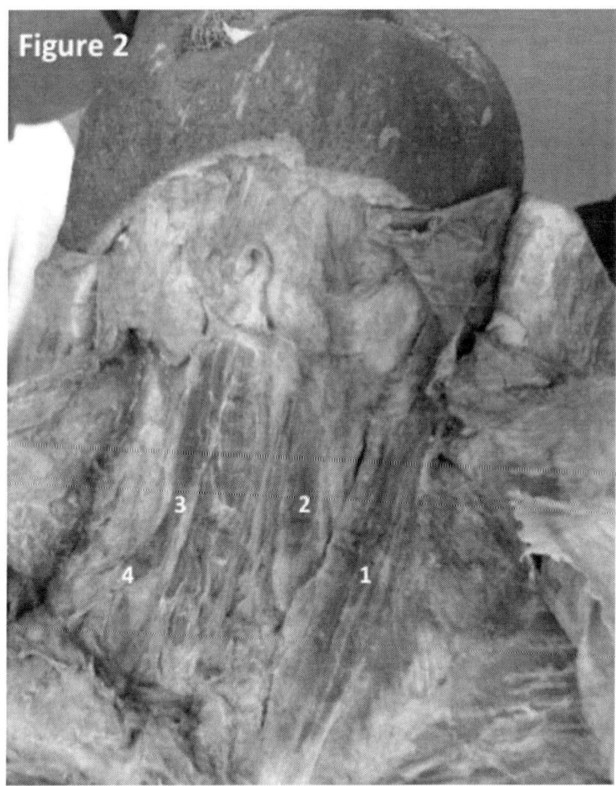

Figure 2. The skin, subcutanous tissue and platymsa have been dissected free to reveal the underlying strap muscles of the neck. Sternocleidomastoid muscle (1) is visible on the left side of the neck obliquely covering the origin of the sternohyoid muscle (2). On the right side, the sternocleidomastoid muscle has been cut and reflected to expose the sternohyoid (2), superior belly of omohyoid (3) and inferior belly of omohyoid (4).

There are two capsules surrounding the thyroid gland. A dense condensation of pre-tracheal fascia forms the outer (false) capsule. The inner true capsule is a thin, fibrous membrane that encapsulates the gland and separates it from surrounding structures. The false capsule also invests the parathyroid glands, firmly applying them to the posterior surface of each lobe.

Therefore, they are at risk of inadvertent injury or excision during thyroidectomy. The gland has two lateral lobes that are connected at their lower thirds [7] by a bridge of tissue - the isthmus (Figure 6).

The isthmus is approximately 2cm in length and 4-6 mm thick. It is constant in position anterior to the second, third and fourth tracheal cartilages where it is firmly applied by fibrous connective tissue.

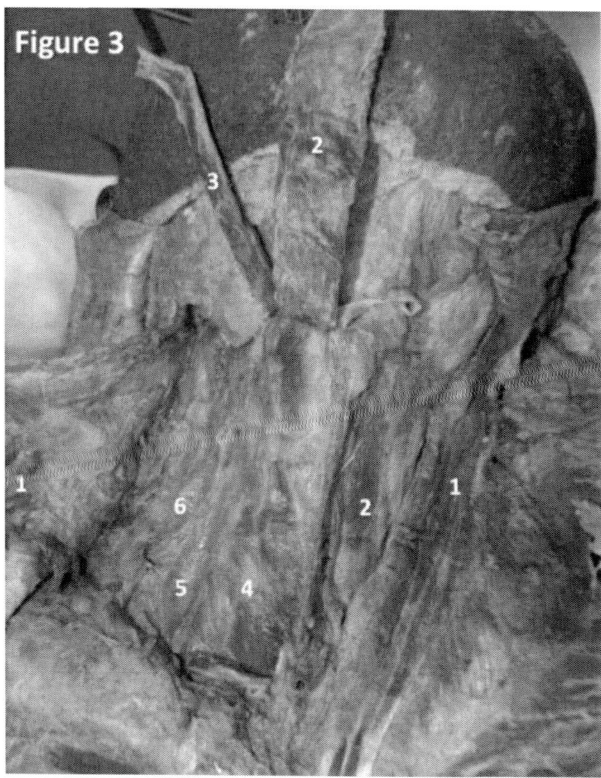

Figure 3. Deeper dissection in the neck. On the left, sternocleidomastoid muscle (1) is visible obliquely covering the origin of sternohyoid (2). On the right side, the sternohyoid (2) and omohyoid (3) have been cut and reflected cephalad to expose the underlying sternothyroid muscle (4). The sternocleidomastoid has been cut and reflected laterally to reveal the carotid artery (5) and internal jugular vein (6) both within the carotid sheath.

In his original paper, Sir James Berry [8] described the suspensory (lateral thyrohyoid) ligament as "*a band of connective tissue that passes from the inner back part of the lateral lobe upward to the cricoid cartilage*" (Figure 7). More recently, Leow et al. [9] demonstrated on 50 cadaveric dissections that there was a more extensive attachment, from the inferior cornu of the thyroid cartilage spanning infero-medially onto the tracheal wall, and even crossing the midline in 8% of cases. This ligament is important from a clinical standpoint because in instances where the thyroid lobes become enlarged, the fixation at this point keeps the gland immobile, thereby determining the final lie of the enlarged gland [10] (i.e. whether it extends retrosternally or remains within the neck).

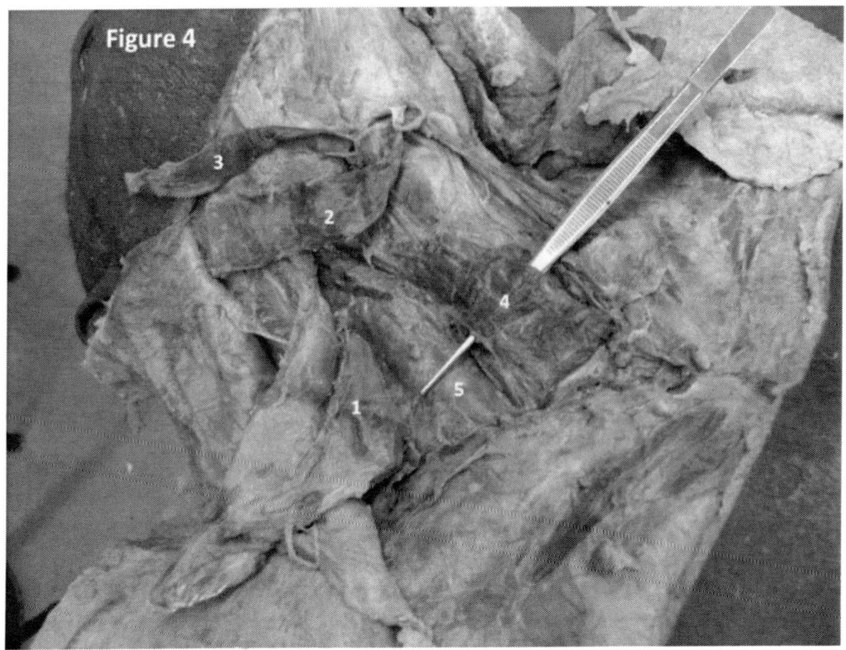

Figure 4. Neck dissection in a cadaver. On the right, the sternohyoid (2) and omohyoid (3) have been cut and reflected cephalad to allow the dissecting forceps to be passed beneath sternothyroid muscle (4). The sternocleidomastoid (1) has been cut and reflected laterally, allowing the tip of the forceps to lie on the carotid sheath (5).

The anatomic course of the recurrent laryngeal nerve (RLN) at this point is of extreme surgical importance (Figure 10). As it ascends in the trachea-oesophageal groove, the RLN passes just postero-lateral to the lateral thyro-hyoid ligament [9-11]. The RLN then travels cephalad for a mean distance of 1.9mm before entering the larynx beneath the inferior constrictor [9].

Consequently, the RLN is particularly prone to iatrogenic injury at this point. Based on the location of the RLN, running lateral to the ligament of Berry [9-11], Naraynsingh et al. [10] advocated early division of the ligament close to the trachea as one means of RLN preservation. However, it is important to remember that there may be great variability in anatomy, especially on the right side of the neck [12]. When Sunada et al. [12] examined the course of 46 nerves in patients undergoing thyroidectomy, they located the RLN lateral to the ligament in 54% of cases - as expected. But they found the RLN posterior to the ligament in the trachea-esophageal groove in 37% of cases; it actually pierced the ligament in 7%; and in 2% the nerve was not visible at this level because a non-recurrent laryngeal nerve was present [12].

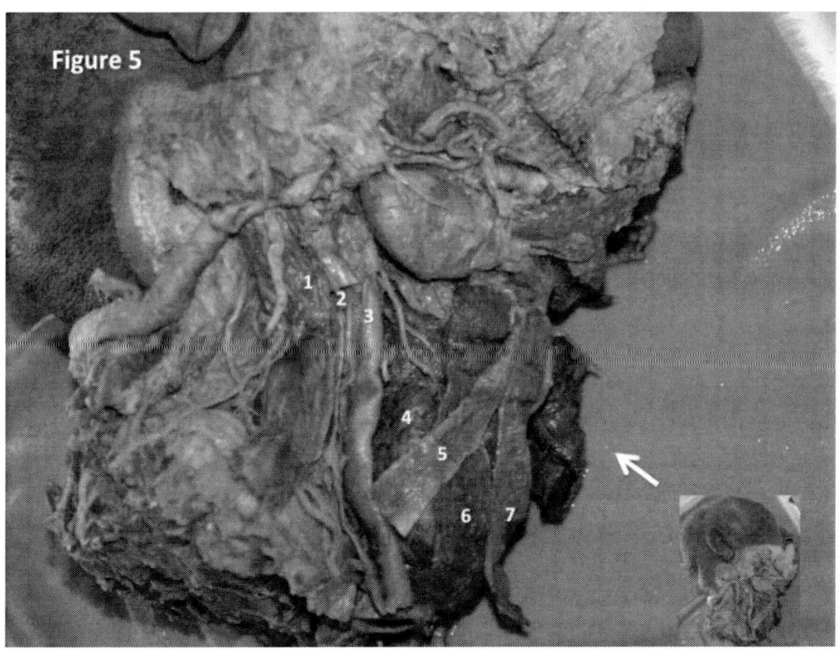

Figure 5. Dissection of the neck in a cadaveric specimen (inset). The sternocleido-mastoid (1) is reflected laterally to maximize exposure of the (transected) internal jugular vein (2), carotid artery (3) and upper pole of the right thyroid lobe (3). The superior belly of omohyoid (5), sternohyoid (6) and sternohyoid (7) are seen covering the thyroid gland anteriorly.

Preservation of the RLN is important because it is the sole supply to all intrinsic muscles of the larynx – except the cricothyroid. Among these, the posterior cricoarytenoid is the only muscle to abduct the vocal cords.

Therefore, unilateral RLN injury allows the ipsilateral vocal cord to assume a cadaveric (adducted) position, producing hoarseness and dysphonia [13, 14]. Bilateral injury is devastating because both cords are adducted, producing airway obstruction [15, 16]. The lateral lobes are roughly conical in shape, approximately measuring 4cm in length, 2cm in breadth and 3cm in thickness. They lie on either side of the trachea with their long axes in a cranio-caudal plane and their apices projecting slightly supero-laterally (Figure 6). The upper pole extends to the junction of middle and upper third of the thyroid cartilage [7]. The lower pole extends caudally to the level of the fifth or sixth tracheal rings [7]. The lateral lobes lie in a gutter that is bounded medially by the inferior constrictor, thyroid cartilage, cricoid cartilage, trachea and cervical oesophagus (Figures 6, 10).

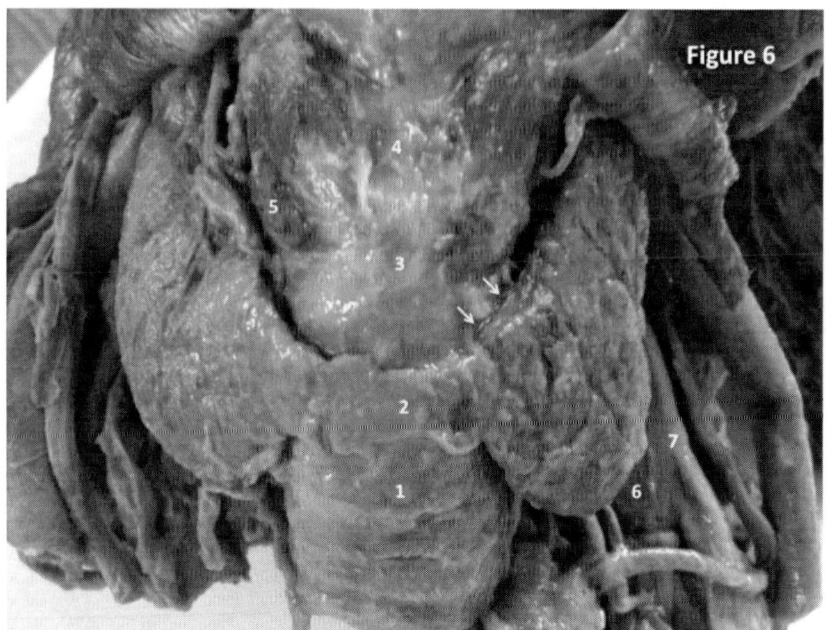

Figure 6. Cadaveric dissection of the thyroid gland in situ. The isthmus (2) is seen connecting both lateral lobes at their lower thirds. The isthmus straddles the trachea (1) in the midline with the lateral lobes reaching posteriorly and laterally, coming to lie in the para-tracheal gutter. In this position, the lateral lobes are related medially to the trachea (1) cricoid caritlage (3), larynx (4) and oesophagus posteriorly (not visible in this photograph). White arrows indicate the position of the lateral thyrohyoid ligament of Berry just caudal to the cricothryoid muscle (5). The scalenus anterior muscle (6) is also seen with inferior thyroid artery (7) ascending on its surface.

The RLN lies in the trachea-oesophageal groove as it courses cephalad. It is at risk of injury or inadvertent transection during mobilization of the lateral lobes.

Figure 11 demonstrates the boundaries of the para-tracheal gutter within which the lateral lobes rest. The lateral wall of this gutter is formed by the sternocleidomastoid and underlying carotid sheath.

Although firmly connected to the trachea and larynx by the lateral thyrohyoid ligaments, the postero-lateral aspects of the lateral lobes lie loosely within thin areolar tissue in the para-tracheal gutter.

This is important surgically as it forms a false capsule where many surgeons choose to commence their dissection to mobilize the gland during a classic thyroidectomy.

The posterior layer of deep cervical fascia forms the floor of the gutter.

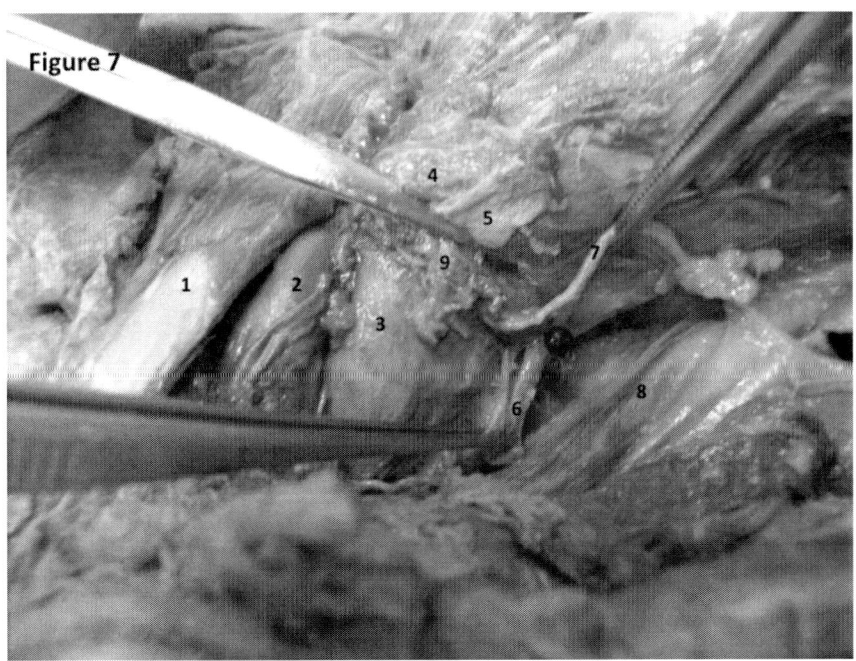

Figure 7. Anterolateral view of a cadaveric neck from the left. Skin, platysma and anterior cervical fascia have been removed. The right sternohyoid muscle (1) and right carotid artery (2) are seen. The trachea (3) is being tented anteriorly in the neck because the middle forceps are forcefully retracting the left lateral lobe of the thyroid (4) anteriorly and over to the right. This allows the thyrohyoid ligament of Berry (5) to be artificially pulled antero-laterally so that it is visible from behind as it runs from the postero-medial part of the thyroid lobe to the cricoid cartilage. Behind the lateral lobe, the recurrent laryngeal nerve (6) can be seen running in the tracheo-esophageal groove. The inferior thyroid artery (7) can be seen taking its characteristic downward turn, leaving the scalenus anterior muscle (8). An important surgical landmark indicated by the black pin is the point at which the inferior thyroid artery crosses the recurrent laryngeal nerve – often used as a landmark to identify the superior parathyroid gland (9).

There are two notable variations with clinical significance that may be present: a tubercle of Zuckerkandl and a pyramidal lobe.

The pyramidal lobe is a projection of thyroid tissue that originates from a base at the upper part of the isthmus or adjacent parts of the lateral lobes (Figure 12) and then projects cranially for variable distances, potentially reaching as high as the hyoid bone (Figure 13) [7].

The pyramidal lobe is a vestigial remnant of the thyroglossal duct that formed during the embryonic stage of development.

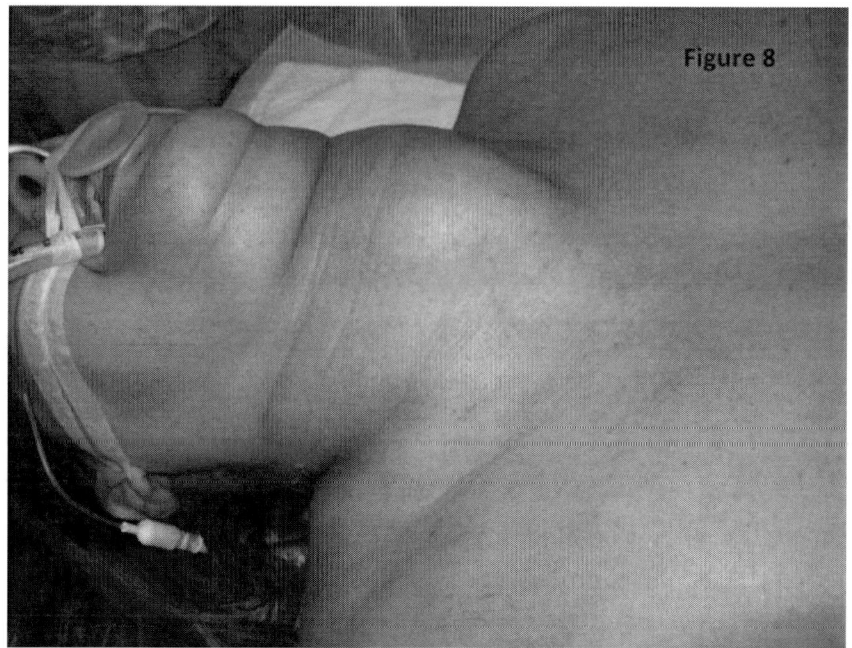

Figure 8. Photograph of a patient on the operating table being prepared for thryoidectomy. Because the isthmus is held firmly in place by the ligament of Berry, the enlarged left upper pole is pushed cranially (cephalization of the gland) accounting for the full-ness at the sub-mandibular region.

This explains why it is in the midline extending toward the middle of the hyoid bone. The pyramidal lobe is inconstant, but tends to be present in disease states where the entire gland becomes hyperplastic such as Grave's disease or Hashimoto's thyroiditis.

From a clinical standpoint, it is surgically important because the remnant tissues may undergo hypertrophy post-thyroidectomy.

The Tubercle of Zuckerkandl is a projection of thyroid tissue that extends from the posterior part of the lateral lobe(s) (Figure 14).

Although Otto Madelung is credited with its discovery [17], it was Emil Zuckerkandl who gave the first detailed description in 1902 and named it the *processus posterior glandulae thyreoideae* [18].

Several investigators have observed this structure at thyroidectomies [17, 19-21] and at autopsies [18, 22-24]. They report a Tubercle of Zuckerkandl being present in 55% [19] to 66% [17] of unselected individuals.

When present, it is usually a unilateral finding and a marker for a co-existent pyramidal lobe [20].

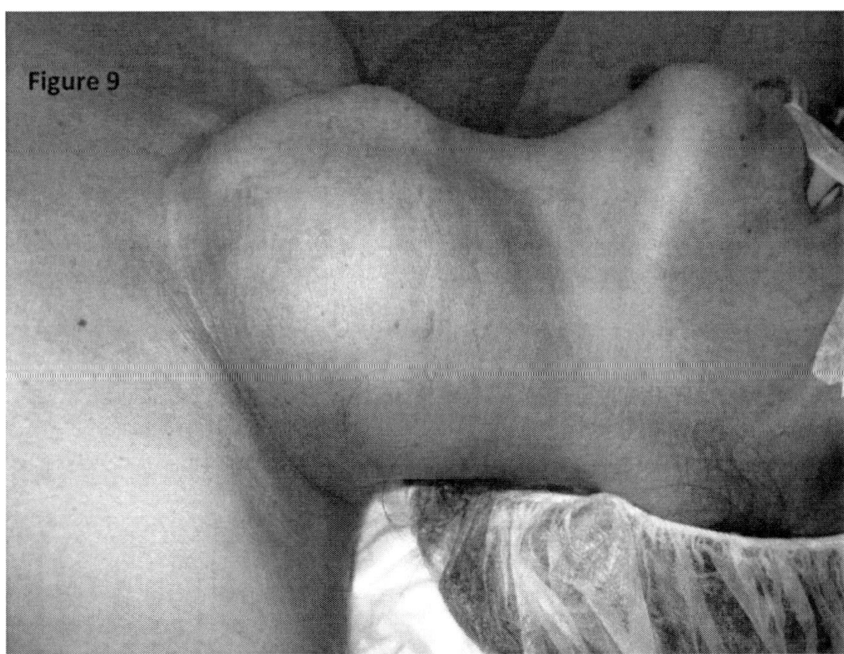

Figure 9. Photograph of a patient on the operating table being prepared for thryoidectomy. Because the isthmus is held firmly in place by the ligament of Berry, the enlarged lower poles are pushed caudally. In this patient, the goitre fills the supra-sternal area and then dives into the superior mediastinum – but the sub-mandibular region is not full because there has been no cephalization of the gland in this case.

Gurleyik et al. [17] prospectively evaluated 160 lateral lobes during routine thyroidectomies and reported that there was a predilection for right-sided tubercles: 61% on the right, 38% on the left and bilateral in 25%.

The tubercles vary widely in size. This prompted Pellizio et al. [22] to propose a four-tiered classification: Grade 0 - unrecognizable; Grade I - thick lateral edge of gland <0.5cm, Grade II - tubercle 0.5-1cm, Grade III - tubercle >1cm. It is a useful anatomic classification but has little clinical application. Yet, a Tubercle of Zuckerkandl is clinically important for three reasons.

Firstly, after a thyroidectomy thyroidal tissue within a remnant tubercle may be the focus of persistent endocrine function and/or recurrence from glandular regeneration. Therefore, surgeons should be aware of the potential for this to exist and they should perform a deliberate search for the Tubercle of Zuckerkandl to ensure complete excision.

Secondly, the Tubercle of Zuckerkandl can facilitate RLN identification [19-24].

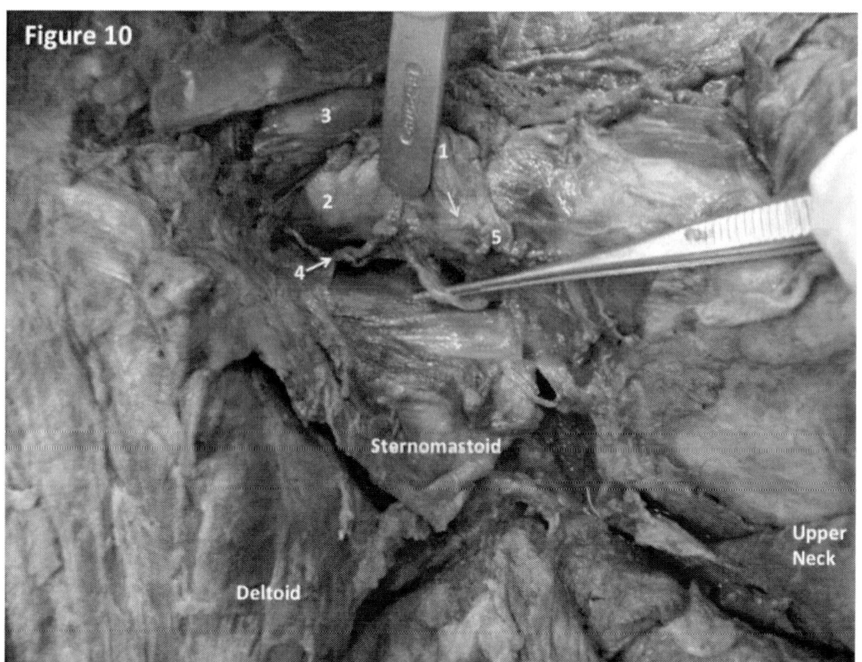

Figure 10. View of the left side of the neck in a dissected cadaver specimen. The left lateral lobe of thyroid (1) is reflected antero-medially, so pulling the trachea (2) anteriorly and over toward the right carotid artery (3). This mobilizes the recurrent laryngeal nerve (4) out of the tracheo-esophageal groove as it runs cephalad (to the right of the photograph) to approach the Ligament of Berry (yellow arrow). The Ligament of Berry in this photograph is artificially mobilized antero-laterally along with the lateral lobe of the thyroid. The superior thyroid artery (5) can also be seen superior and medial to the Ligament of Berry.

It does this by "pointing toward" the junction where the inferior thyroid artery crosses over the RLN just infero-lateral to the ligament of Berry (Figure 7). It is not difficult to appreciate, therefore, that this last 2-3cm of the extra-laryngeal course of the RLN is the point of greatest potential for nerve injury, especially when an enlarged tubercle obscures this part of the nerve course [19-24].

Finally, there are recognized variations that surgeons must be aware of. Normally the RLN is found in the trachea-oesophageal groove medial (also described as posterior) to the tubercle in 93% [21] to 94% [17, 19] of cases. The tubercle may occasionally be wedged between the RLN and the trachea-oesophageal groove. In this case, the RLN lies lateral (also described as anterior) to the tubercle of Zuckerkandl.

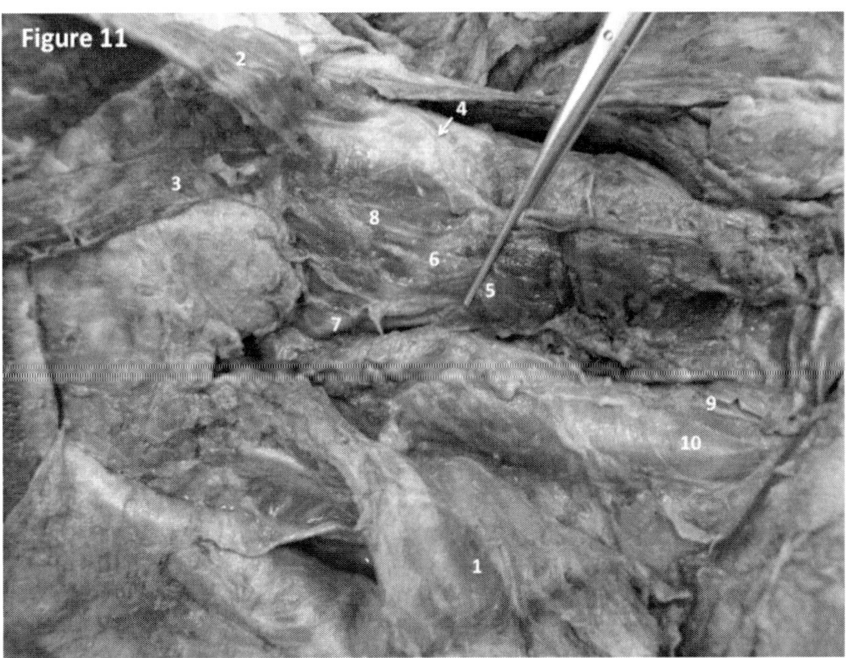

Figure 11. A view of the cadaveric neck dissection from the right side of the neck demonstrating the boundaries of the para-tracheal gutter within which the lateral lobes rest. The sternocleidomastoid muscle (1) is cut and reflected laterally. The thyrohyoid (2) and omohyoid (3) have been cut and reflected cranially. On the medial aspect the lateral lobes are in contact with inferior constrictor, thyroid cartilage (4), (5) oblique line of the thyroid carilage (6), cricoid cartilage, trachea and cervical oesophagus (not seen in this photograph). Laterally, the lobes are in contact with sternocleidomastoid muscle (1) and carotid artery (9) with internal jugular vein (10) both wrapped the carotid sheath. Note the superior thyroid artery (7) as it descends just posterior to the border of thyrohyoid muscle (8).

This variation is found in 6% [17, 19] to 7% [21] of individuals with a tubercle. This anterior location is a dangerous variation as it places the RLN at high risk of iatrogenic injury during dissection.

Blood Supply

Two pairs of arteries consistently supply arterial blood to the thyroid gland. The superior thyroid arteries arise as the first branches from the external carotid artery just below the greater horn of the hyoid bone [7].

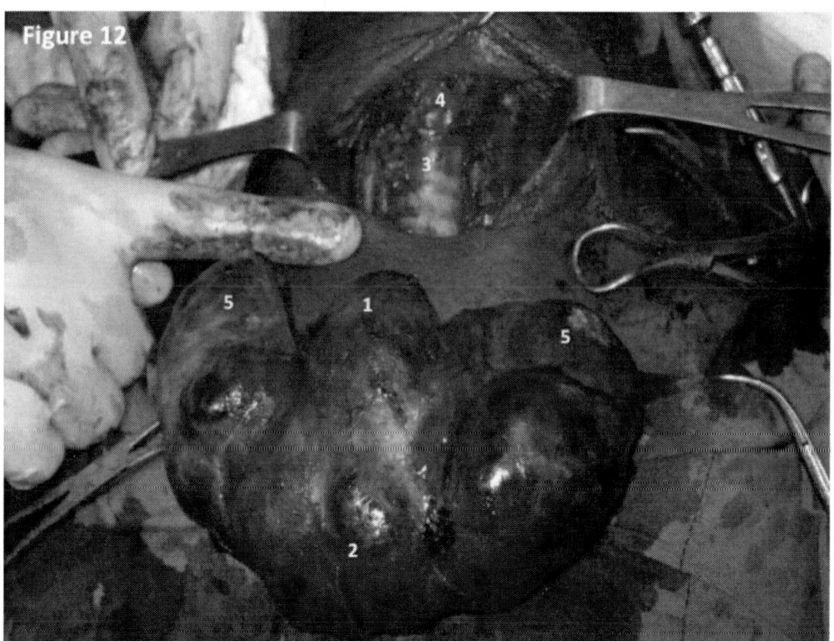

Figure 12. Intra-operative picture of a patient post total thyroidectomy. The specimen has been excised en bloc and is placed on the patient's chest to show the orientation of the gland. A thick pyramidal lobe (1) can be seen arising from the isthmus (2). The extent of neck dissection demonstrates the course of the pyramidal lobe, passing cephalad in the midline over the trachea (3) up to the level of the thyroid cartilage (4). The lateral lobes (5) have also extended upward into the neck in the process of glandular cephalization.

The artery descends to the upper pole of the thyroid, supplying the omohyoid, sternothyroid and sterohyoid muscles as it passes deep to them (Figure 15). As it approaches the upper pole, the superior thyroid artery breaks into three un-named branches [7]: one supplying the upper part of the isthmus, a second passing posteriorly to supply the posteromedial part of upper lobe, and a third passing antero-laterally to supply the anterior part of the upper lobe.

The branches anastomose with their fellow on the opposite sides and the inferior thyroid artery. In its course, the superior thyroid artery is closely related to the external branch of the superior laryngeal nerve (EBSLN). The EBSLN descends on the surface of the inferior constrictor to pierce and supply cricothyroid [25, 26] (Figure 15).

The EBSLN provides the only motor supply to cricothyroid. Through its action to elongate and tense the vocal cords, it plays an important role in phonation and determination of pitch.

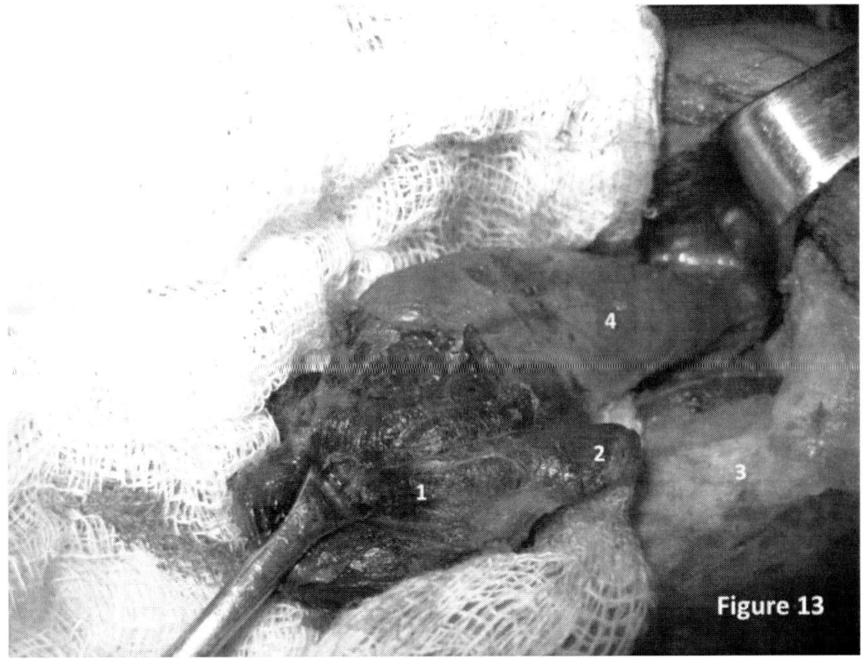

Figure 13. Intra-operative picture during a right hemi-thyroidectomy. The isthmus (1) has been divided as the initial step of a retrograde thyroidectomy. An ischemic pyramidal lobe (2) can be seen extending upward in the midline over the trachea (3). Forceful retraction of the upper skin flap with a Langenbeck's retractor reveals the upper pole of the right lobe (4).

The course of the EBSLN is highly variable. Several authors have attempted to define the variations based on the relationships between the EBSLN and the superior thyroid artery. Cernea et al. [27] proposed a classification based on the distance from the upper pole at which the superior thyroid artery crosses the EBSLN (Figure 15). This is a clinically relevant classification as it can stratify patient risk for EBSLN injury. Type 1 refers to the situation in which the artery crosses the EBSLN >1cm above the upper pole. This is present in 23% [28] to 43% [27] of cases. Type 2a variations, where the artery crosses the EBSLN <1cm above the upper pole, is present in 37% [27] to 60% [28] of persons. Type 2b variation, where the artery crosses over the EBSLN below the upper pole of thyroid, is seen in 18% [28] to 20% [27] of individuals. These patients have a very high risk of inadvertent EBSLN injury during ligation of the upper pole pedicle. Although Cernea's classification [27] may stratify nerve injury risk in individuals with normal thyroid glands, the classification may be misleading when a goiter is present.

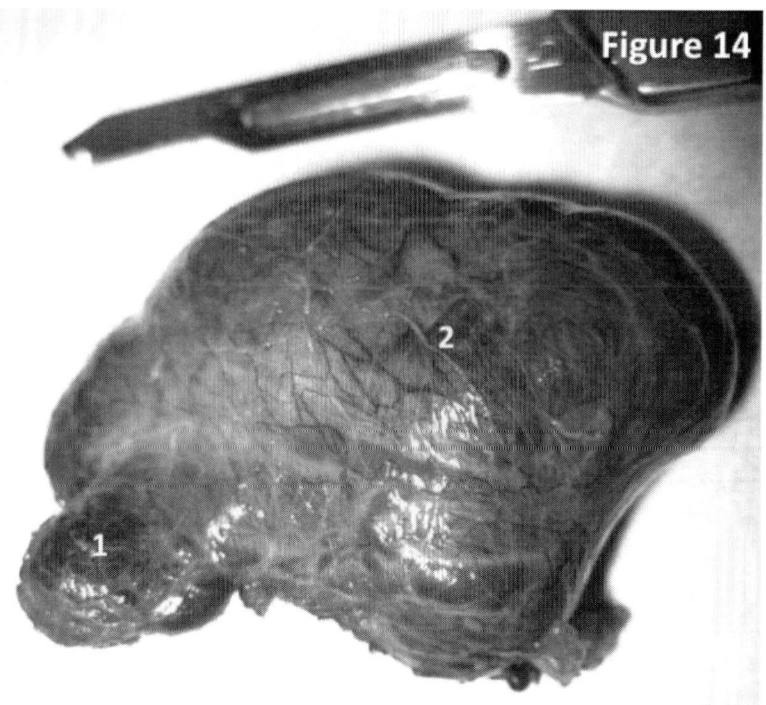

Figure 14. An excised specimen after right hemi-thyroidectomy (viewed from the lateral aspect). A large Tubercle of Zuckerkandl (1) can be seen at the postero-lateral aspect of the right lateral lobe (2).

Due to the gland's firm fixation by the lateral thyrohyoid ligaments, any pathology at the upper poles will result in "cephalization" of the gland (upward extension of an enlarged lateral lobe due to fixity by the ligament of Berry). In this instance, the basis of Cernea's classification [27] - the point at which the superior thyroid artery crosses the EBSLN - now has an abnormal relationship that makes the classification ineffective.

The inferior thyroid arteries originate from the thyrocervical trunk (thyroid axis) – a thick, short branch that comes off the first part of the subclavian artery (figure 16). They ascend upward obliquely on the surface of the scalenus anterior muscle, between the vertebral artery (behind) and the internal jugular vein (in front). At a level just below the carotid tubercle and at about the level of omohyoid tendon, the inferior thyroid artery turns medially. It passes behind the carotid artery within its sheath and takes a characteristic downward turn to reach the posterior surface of the lateral lobe (Figures 7 and 16).

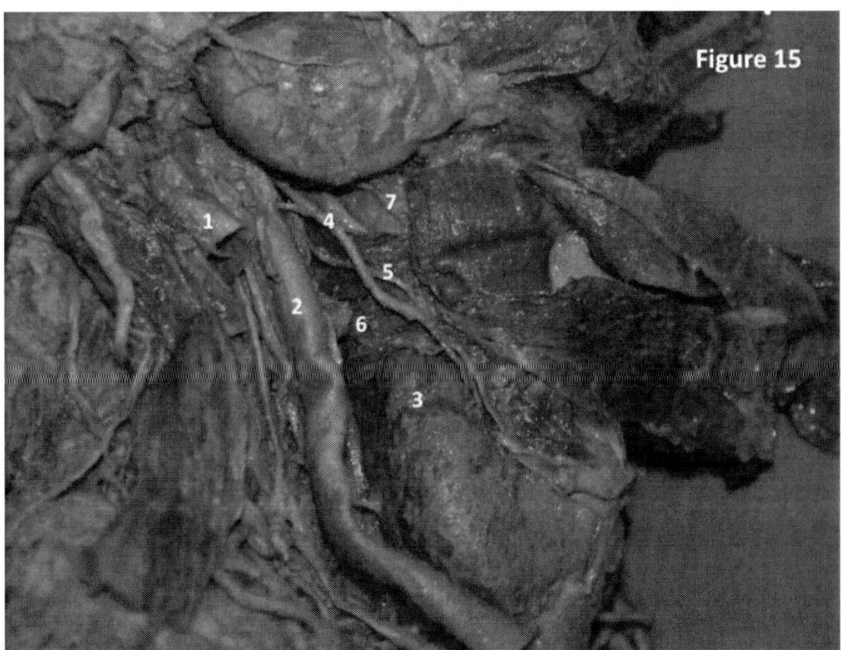

Figure 15. Cadaveric dissection of the neck with the strap muscles retracted antero-medially to expose the internal jugular vein (1), external carotid artery (2) and the lateral lobe of the thyroid gland (3). The superior thryoid artery (4) is seen arising as the first branch of the external carotid artery (2). It courses antero-inferiorly lying on the inferior constrictor muscle (6) and traveling with the external branch of the superior laryngeal nerve (5) to reach the upper pole of the thyroid (3). Here the artery can be seen breaking into three branches that permeate the thyroid substance antero-medially, posterolaterally and at the isthmus. The internal branch of the superior laryngeal nerve (7) is also visible beneath the parotid gland.

Here, the inferior thyroid artery usually crosses over the RLN, but great variability exits. When Sunada et al. [12] studied the course of 46 RLNs in patients at thyroidectomy, a normal relationship was found in 61% of cases. However, the RLN passed through branches of the inferior thyroid artery in 24% of cases, anterior to the artery in 9% and in 2% of cases there was no relationship with RLN due to the presence of a non-recurrent RLN [12].

Inconsistently, a thyroidea ima is encountered in 0.5-6% of persons [29]. When present, it has several potential origins (Figure 17). Gruber et al. [30] reported that in a series of 90 cases, the commonest origins were innominate artery followed by aortic arch, common carotid and internal thoracic arteries, transverse scapular and suprascapular arteries. It ascends in front of the trachea in the midline to reach the inferior surface of the isthmus in the midline.

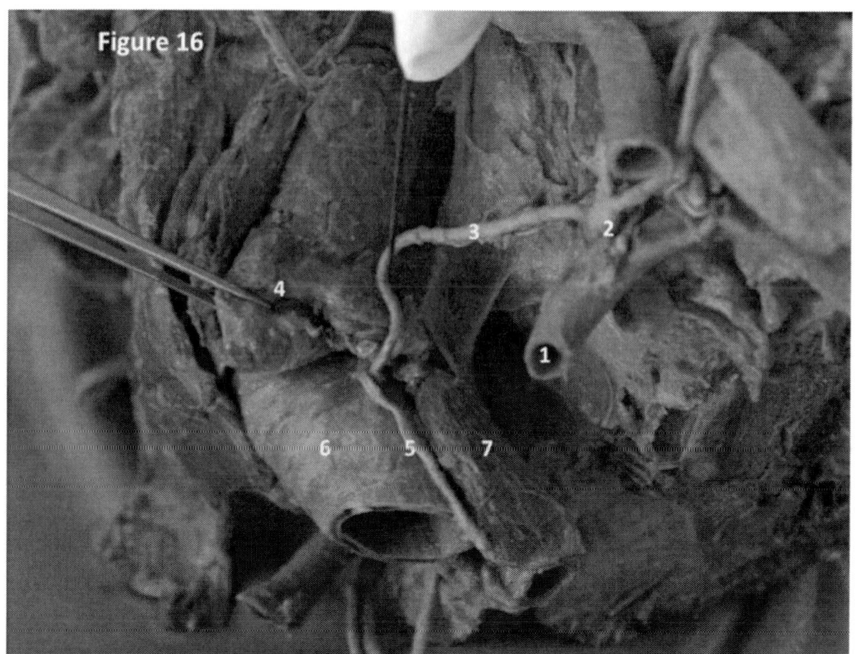

Figure 16. Anterolateral dissection of a cadaveric neck demonstrating the subclavian artery (1) and the thyrocervical trunk (2). The inferior thyroid artery (3) is seen originating from the thyrocervical trunk. The inferior thyroid artery travels cephalad for a short distance before taking the characteristic infre-medial turn to reach the posterior part of the lateral lobe (4). At this point, it is closely related to the recurrent laryngeal nerve (5) that courses cephalad in the groove between the trachea (6) and oesophagus (7). In this case the recurrent laryngeal nerve is seen crossing in front of the inferior thyroid artery.

In this course, it may be at risk for inadvertent injury during tracheostomies or sub-total thyroidectomy.

After reaching the gland the arteries divide into multiple large un-named branches that ramify on the glandular surface beneath the true capsule, forming an extensive superficial network with free anastomoses in the gland. From this superficial network, multiple smaller arteries permeate into the substance of the gland forming rich anastomotic capillary networks around the follicles.

Venules coalesce to form a plexus of veins beneath the capsule that drain into three pairs of named veins. The superior thyroid veins exit the upper pole and eventually empty into the upper part of the internal jugular vein. Similarly, the inferior thyroid veins leave the lower pole by traveling in the inferior pedicle.

The inferior parathyroid glands and the thymus originate from the third ryngeal pouch and they migrate together toward the anterior mediastinum. ially, the inferior parathyroid separates and comes to rest near the lower of the thyroid, but in 26% of individuals [32] they may rest in ectopic ations anywhere along the path of thymic descent into the anterior diastinum [33]. Up to 60% of ectopic glands are just infero-lateral to the er pole of the thyroid [37]. Other less common rests are beside the aortic , along the hypoglossal nerve, in the aorto-pulmonary window or in the cardium [37-40]. Although there are usually four parathyroid glands, er-numerary glands may exist in 5% of cases [32]. This is believed to be to improper separa-ion of the pharyngeal pouches during embryogenesis.

When present, the supernumerary glands are found near the lower poles of thyroid, in the thymus or near the jugulo-carotid axis [32].

od Supply

In 68% of cases, the upper branch of the inferior thyroid artery supplies superior parathyroid gland [41]. Occasionally the superior parathyroid may receive significant supply from a posterior branch of the superior thyroid ry [42]. The inferior thyroid artery also supplies the inferior parathyroids in 80% of cases [41], also taking branches of the inferior thyroid artery with n when they are found in ectopic locations. However, ectopic glands in the iastinum tend to have additional supply from the internal thoracic artery or ctly from the aorta.

Conclusion

Surgeons who perform operations on the thyroid or parathyroid glands t be familiar with the anatomy of these glands and the anatomic variations are common with these organs.

References

Giddings, A. E. The History of Thyroidectomy. *J. Royal Soc. Med.* 1998; 91(33): 3-6.

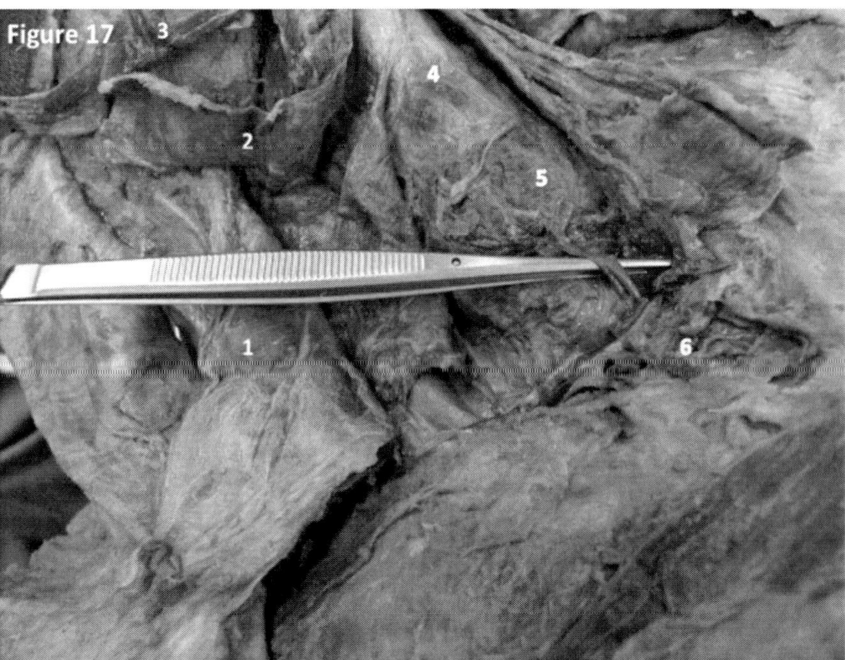

Figure 17. Dissection of the anterior neck in a cadaver. The sternomastoid (1), sterno-hyoid (2) and omohyoid (3) muscles on the right are reflected to expose the upper trachea (4) and the isthmus (5). The surgical forceps are passed behind the thyroidea ima that originates deep in the thorax. The thyroidea ima can be seen exiting the superior mediastinum behind the sternal notch (6), ascending in the midline in front of the trachea to reach the inferior surface of the isthmus in the midline.

The left vein descends to empty into the left innominate trunk and the right vein passes inferiorly and laterally across the innominate artery to empty into the right innominate vein just at its junction with the superior vena cava.

The short middle thyroid vein leaves the lower part of the lateral lobe to empty into the lower part of the internal jugular vein. This vein is encountered and ligated early in the classic approach to thyroidectomy during mobilization of the lateral lobe.

Lymphatic Drainage

Several lymphatic channels surround the follicles and coalesce beneath the true capsule to form collecting trunks. Lymphatic channels follow the venous drainage of the thyroid gland.

From the upper isthmus and supero-medial parts of the lobes, lymphatic channels drain toward the pre-laryngeal "Delphian" nodes and onward to the digastric nodes. These channels drain a pyramidal lobe when present.

Lymphatics from lateral parts of the upper lobe follow the superior thyroid vein, passing behind the sternohyoid to empty into the mid-jugular and retropharyngeal nodes. Lymphatic channels from the lower part of the isthmus and the lower parts of the lateral lobe follow the inferior thyroid veins, eventually draining into antero-superior mediastinal nodes around the innominate veins. Lymphatic channels from the postero-medial aspect of the lobes travel to the tracheo-esophageal groove and eventually empty into nodal chains traveling along the RLN.

Nerve Supply

The gland is innervated by the autonomic nervous systems, but its physiological significance remains to be fully elucidated. Sympathetic supply is derived from the cervical ganglia and the fibres enter the gland by traveling along the blood vessels. Parasympathetic supply is derived from the vagus nerve and travels to the thyroid through branches of the laryngeal nerves.

Parathyroid Glands

There are 4 parathyroid glands, each weighing approximately 20-40gms, plastered to the posterior aspect of the thyroid near the upper and lower poles. The glands are encapsulated and have a smooth surface, differentiating them from the lobulated thyroid. However, the oxyphil cells impart a characteristic tan-yellow color that makes them appear similar to fat in the living patient. This may present difficulty for the surgeon when attempting to identify the gland intra-operatively. During the fifth week of embryogenesis, the superior glands migrate from the 4th pharyngeal pouch together with the ultimo-branchial body [31]. The cells fuse with the posterior part of the thyroid and form the superior parathyroid and the para-follicular C cells respectively. The location of the superior parathyroid gland is relatively constant. It is characteristically found on the postero-lateral surface of the upper pole just above the point of intersection of the inferior thyroid artery and recurrent laryngeal nerve (figure 18). This is an important surgical landmark when trying to identify the superior parathyroid intra-operatively.

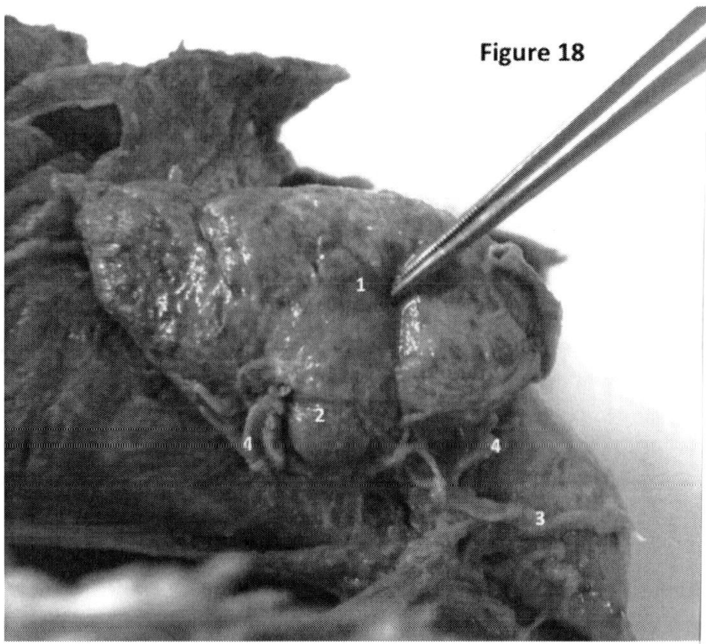

Figure 18. Cadaveric neck viewed from the right side. The forceps are p lateral lobe of the thyroid (1) in order to retract it anteriorly. By reflectir lobe, the parathyroid gland (2) becomes visible on the posterior surface The recurrent laryngeal nerve (3) is visible at the tracheo-esophageal gr cephalad. Several branches of the inferior thyroid artery (4) are seen co anteriorly to supply the posterior surface of the gland.

In 18% of individuals, a superior parathyroid gland may be location [32]. The commoner locations for an ectopic superior g the tracheo-esophageal groove or behind the pharynx / oesophag

Alternatively, the ultimobranchial bodies may fail to se embryonic development causing the superior glands becon embedded within the thyroid parenchyma as an intra-thyroid par [31, 33].

Most intra-thyroid glands are detected when searching for glands in operations for hyperparathyroidism. Goodman et al. that 0.7% parathyroids were embedded within thyroid retrospectively evaluated 10,000 patients who had neck e primary hyperparathyroidism. Most authorities accept an incid 0.2% [32] and 1.4% [35], although a single study from Russia re to 22.7% of parathyroid adenomas embedded within the thyroid

[2] Halsted, W. S. The Operative Story of Goitre. *John Hopkins Hosp. Rep.* 1920; 19: 71-257.

[3] Gemsenjäger, E. Milestones in European Thyroidology: Theodor Kocher (1841-1917). *Eurothyroid.* [Available online http://www.eurothyroid.com/about/met/kocher.html] Accessed April 25, 2014.

[4] Dunhill, T. P. Operations for exophthalmic Goitre. *Br. J. Surg.* 1919; 7: 195-210.

[5] Lahey, F. H. Exposure of recurrent laryngeal nerves in Thyroid Operations. *Surg. Gynaecol. Obstet.* 1944; 78: 293.

[6] Zambudio, A. R., Rodriquez, J., Riquelme, J., Soria, T., Canteras, M., Parrilla, P. Prospective Study of Postoperative Complications after Total Thyroidectomy for Multinodular Goiters by Surgeons with Experience in Endocrine Surgery. *Ann. Surg.* 2004; 240(1): 18-25.

[7] Grays Anatomy. Editors T. Pickering Pick and Robert Hoeden. *The Complete Gray's Anatomy.* 16th edition Edition published 2003 by Merchant Book Company. Eas Molesey, KT8 2WZ. Chapter: The Ductless Glands. Page 1162-1164.

[8] Berry, James. *Diseases of the Thyroid Gland and Their Surgical Treatment.* 1901. London: 7-8.

[9] Leow, C. K., Webb, A. J. The lateral thyroid ligament of Berry. *Int. Surg.* 1988; 38(1): 75-78.

[10] Naraynsingh, V., Cawich, S. O., Maharaj, R., Dan, D. Retrograde Thyroidectomy: A Technique for Visualization and Preservation of the External Branch of Superior Laryngeal Nerve. *International J. Surg. Case Repo.* 2014: 5(3): 122-125.

[11] Sasou, S., Nakamura, S., Kurihara, H. Suspensory ligament of Berry: its relationship to recurrent laryngeal nerve and anatomic examination of 24 autopsies. *Head Neck.* 1988; 20(8): 695-698.

[12] Sunada, H., Tilakeratne, S., De Silva, K. P. Surgical anatomy of the recurrent laryngeal nerve; a cross-sectional descriptive study. *Galle Med. J.* 2010; 15(1): 14-16.

[13] Zakaria, H. M., Al Awad, N. A., Al Kreedes, A. S., Al Mulhim, A. M. A., Al-Sharway, M. A., Abdul Hadi, M., Sayyah, A. A. Recurrent Laryngeal Nerve Injury in Thyroid Surgery. *Oman Med. J.* 2011; 26(1): 34–38.

[14] Eisele, D. W. Intraoperative electrophysiologic monitoring of the recurrent laryngeal nerve. *Laryngoscope* 1996; 106(4): 443-449.

[15] Dimov, R. S., Doikov, I. J., Mitov, F. S., Deenichin, G. P., Yovchev, I. J. Intraoperative identification of recurrent laryngeal nerves in thyroid

surgery by electrical stimulation. *Folia Med.* (Plovdiv) 2001; 43(4): 10-13.

[16] Marcus, B., Edwards, B., Yoo, S., Byrne, A., Gupta, A., Kandrevas, J., et al. Recurrent laryngeal nerve monitoring in thyroid and parathyroid surgery: the University of Michigan experience. *Laryngoscope* 2003; 113(2): 356-361.

[17] Gurleyik, E., Gurleyik, G. Incidence and Surgical Importance of Zuckerkandl's Tubercle of the Thyroid and Its Relations with Recurrent Laryngeal Nerve. *ISRN Surg.* 2012; 450589: 1-5. doi:10.5402/2012/450589.

[18] Zuckerkandl, E. Die Epithelkörperchen von Didelphys azara nebst Bemerkungen über die Epithelkörperchen des Menschen. *Anatomische Hefte.* 1902; 19(1): 59-84.

[19] Hisham, A. N., Lukman, M. R. Recurrent laryngeal nerve in thyroid surgery: a critical appraisal. *ANZ J. Surg.* 2002; 72(12): 887-889.

[20] Delbridge, L. Total thyroidectomy: the evolution of surgical technique. *ANZ J. Surg.* 2003; 73(9): 761–768.

[21] Gauger, P. G., Delbridge, L. W., Thompson, N. W., Crummer, P., Reeve, T. S. Incidence and importance of the tubercle of Zuckerkandl in thyroid surgery. *Eur. J. Surg.* 2001; 167(4): 249-254.

[22] Pelizzo, M. R., Toniato, A., Gemo, G. Zuckerkandl's tuberculum: an arrow pointing to the recurrent laryngeal nerve (constant anatomical landmark). *J. Am. Coll. Surg.* 1998; 3: 333-336.

[23] Kaisha, W., Wobenjo, A., Saidi, H. Topography of the recurrent laryngeal nerve in relation to the thyroid artery, Zuckerkandl tubercle, and Berry ligament in Kenyans. *Clin. Anat.* 2011; 24: 853–857.

[24] Yalcin, B., Ozan, H. Relationship between the Zuckerkandl's tubercle and entrance point of the inferior laryngeal nerve. *Clin. Anat.* 2007; 20 (6): 640–643.

[25] Finck, C. Laryngeal Dysfunction After Thyroid Surgery: Diagnosis, Evaluation and Treatment. *Acta Chir. Belg.* 2006; 106: 378-387.

[26] Kochilas, X., Bibas, A., Xenellis, J., Anagnostopoulou, S. Surgical anatomy of the external branch of the superior laryngeal nerve and its clinical significance in head and neck surgery. *Clin. Anat.* 2008; 21(2): 99-105.

[27] Cernea, C. R., Ferraz, A. R., Nishio, S., Dutra, A., Hojail, F. C., Dos Santos, L. R. Surgical anatomy of the external branch of the superior laryngeal nerve. *Head Neck.* 1992; 14(5): 380-383.

[28] Ozlugedik, S., Acar, H. I., Apaydin, N., Tekdemir, I., Elhan, A., Comert, A. Surgical anatomy of the external branch of the superior laryngeal nerve. *Clin. Anat.* 2007; 20(4): 387-391.

[29] Saadeh, F. A., Hawi, J. S. The thyroidea ima artery revisited. *Case Rep. Clin. Pract. Rev.,* 2003; 4(1): 16-17.

[30] Gruber, W. Ueber die Arteria thyroidea ima. *Arch. Pathol. Anat. Physiol. Klin. Med.* 1872; 54: 445-484.

[31] Mirilas, P. Lateral congenital anomalies of the pharyngeal apparatus: part I. Normal developmental anatomy (embryogenesis) for the surgeon. *Am. Surg.* 2011; 77(9): 1230-1242.

[32] Lappas, D., Noussios, G., Anagnostis, P., Adamidou, F., Chatzigeorgiou, A., Skandalakis, P. Location, number and morphology of parathyroid glands: results from a large anatomical series. *Anat. Sci. Int.* 2012;87 (3): 160-164. doi: 10.1007/s12565-012-0142-1.

[33] Noussios, G., Anagostis, P., Natsis, K. Ectopic parathyroid glands and their anatomical, clinical and surgical implications. *Exp. Clin. Endocrinol. Diabetes.* 2012; 120(10): 604-10. doi: 10.1055/s-0032-1327628.

[34] Goodman, A., Politz, D., Lopez, J., Norman, J. Intrathyroid parathyroid adenoma: incidence and location-the case against thyroid lobectomy. *Otolaryngol. Head Neck Surg.* 2011; 144: 867-871.

[35] Bahar, G., Feinmesser, R., Joshua, B. Z., et al. Hyperfunctioning intrathyroid parathyroid gland: a potential cause of failure in parathyroidectomy. *Surgery* 2006; 139: 821-826.

[36] Romanchishen, A. F., Matveeva, Z. S. Intrathyroid parathyroid adenomas. *Vestn. Khir. Im. I. I. Grek.* 2007; 166: 40-42.

[37] Gough, I. Reoperative parathyroid surgery: the importance of ectopic location and multigland disease. *ANZ J. Surg.* 2006; 76(12): 1048-1050.

[38] Karvounaris, D. C., Symeonidis, N., Triantafyllou, A., Flaris, N., Sakadamis, A. Ectopic parathyroid adenoma located inside the hypo-glossal nerve. *Head Neck* 2010; 32: 1273-1276.

[39] Arnault, V., Beaulieu, A., Lifante, J. C., et al. Multicenter study of 19 aortopulmonary window parathyroid tumors: the challenge of embryologic origin. *World J. Surg.* 2010; 34: 2211-2216.

[40] Yadav, R., Mohammed, T. L., Neumann, D. R., Mihaljevic, T., Hoschar, A. Case of the season: ectopic parathyroid adenoma in the pericardium: a report of robotically assisted minimally invasive parathyroidectomy. *Semin. Roentgenol.* 2010; 45: 53-56.

[41] Hi, Z. D., Liu, H. W., Dong, H. L., Li, S. C. Preservation of parathyroid glands and their functions during total thyroidectomy. *Chinese J. Otorhin. Head Neck Surg*. 2010; 45(11): 899-903.

[42] Nobori, M., Saiki, S., Tanaka, N., Harihara, Y., Sindo, S., Fujimoto, Y. Blood supply of the parathyroid gland from the superior thyroid artery. *Surg*. 1994; 115(4): 417-423.

In: Thyroidectomy
Editor: Kimberly Rodolfo
ISBN: 978-1-63321-440-8

Chapter 7

Endoscopic and Robotic Thyroidectomy

David Ka-kin Tsui*[*] *and Chung-ngai Tang
Department of Surgery, Pamela Youde Nethersole Eastern Hospital, Chai Wan, Hong Kong, SAR

Abstract

Thyroid surgery is traditionally performed using Kocher incision over the neck for years. With the development of minimal access surgical equipment, there are a variety of surgical methods to achieve thyroid surgery with a good cosmetic result. These include cervical approach by means of minimally invasive video-assisted thyroidectomy using a mini-incision in the neck, or extra-cervical approach by means of remote access via the breast, chest wall and/or axilla. With the use of da Vinci Robotic Surgical System, we would expect this operation to be performed under a steady, magnified and high definition videoscopic view at a higher surgical cost.

In this chapter, we will discuss various methods of endoscopic thyroidectomy. Indication, surgical procedure and potential benefits of each procedure will be highlighted. We will also share our own series of endoscopic and robotic thyroidectomy. The potential complications and special precautions will be discussed as well. We hope our reader will

[*] Corresponding author: Email: drkktsui@gmail.com.

have an overview on endoscopic and robotic thyroidectomy after reading this chapter.

Introduction

Thyroid surgery is one of the commonly performed general surgical operations. In the old days, thyroid surgery was associated with significant morbidity or even mortality. Theodor Kocher (1841-1917) has won the Nobel Prize in Physiology or Medicine in 1909 for "his work on the physiology, pathology and surgery of the thyroid gland". With the better knowledge about thyroid anatomy, thyroid surgery becomes safer over the years. Nowadays, the mortality from thyroid surgery is kept to a minimum.

On the other hand, with the development minimal access surgical equipment, thyroid surgery can be performed with a smaller incision depending on situations. In order to achieve the best cosmetic result, the incision may be placed little away from the neck, or far away (remote incision) at the site which can be covered by clothings.

Development of Minimally Invasive Techniques on Thyroid Surgery

Traditional thyroid surgery involved a neck collar incision [Figure 1]. Although it can provide a good access for surgery, some patients may have hypertrophic or keloid scars after the surgery. The access wound can be minimized by means of a smaller incision while the surgical view is being maintained by videoscopic assistance. Gagner [1] reported the first endoscopic parathyroidectomy in 1996 and Hüscher et al. [2] performed the first video-assisted endoscopic thyroid lobectomy in 1997. Further efforts from other parties were made to perform surgery in a magnified view under videoscopic assistance through a smaller incision (cervical access). On the other hand, another group of surgeons performed thyroid surgery with incision further away from the neck to improve the cosmetic results (extra-cervical or remote access).

Cervical Access

The initial development of cervical access involves a mini-incision in the neck. The pioneer in this technique is Paolo Miccoli from Italy who reported his series of minimally invasive video-assisted thyroidectomy (MIVAT) [3]. This procedure starts with a 15mm incision above the sternal notch. Skin retractors can be used to increase the exposure.

Needlescopic instruments and 30 degree 5mm laparoscope are used for visualization of important structures including the parathyroid glands, the recurrent laryngeal nerve as well as the external branch of superficial laryngeal nerve. Vascular pedicles can be ligated between clips or controlled with ultrasonic sealing devices through this mini-incision. This procedure can be performed under a video-assisted manner without CO_2 insufflation.

The MIVAT procedure is widely practiced in European countries showing comparable results to conventional open surgery. Prospective randomized controlled study between MIVAT and conventional thyroidectomy has shown that the MIVAT procedure may have less postoperative pain and good cosmetic outcome [4].

Cervical endoscopic surgery by incisions over the anterior neck with CO_2 insufflation was also described for the management of small thyroid nodules [5]. Similar to MIVAT, needlescopic instruments, ultrasonic shears and angled laparoscope are used.

In Japan, Shimizu et al. reported his thyroidectomy procedure by the video-assisted neck surgery (VANS) [6]. He starts the procedure with a 1.5cm infraclavicular incision. Blunt finger dissection can be used to develop the subplatysmal flap. Two pieces of Kirschner wire 1.2mm in diameter are inserted horizontally in the subcutaneous layer of the anterior neck. These are then lifted up and fixed to an L-shape pole to create a tent-like working space. The working space is maintained by this special skin lifting device without the needle of CO_2 insufflation.

Two other working ports can be inserted under direct vision. Total lobectomy and prophylactic neck dissection can be performed using this approach [7]. The incisions can be covered by open-neck clothes of patients later.

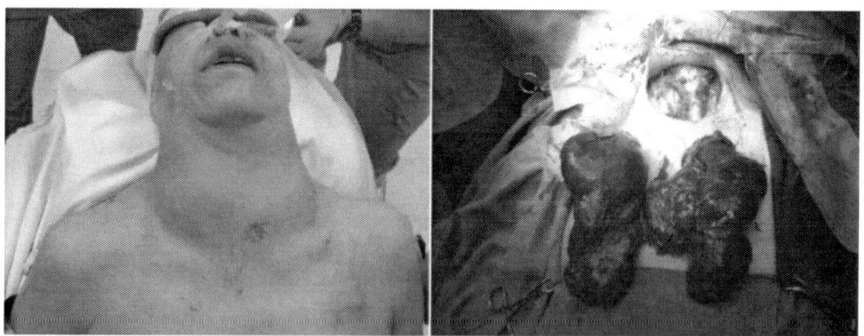

Figure 1. Conventional open thyroidectomy by Kocher incision.

Extra-Cervical Access or Remote Access

In order to perform thyroidectomy without a neck incision, the 'scarless neck' procedure, some surgeons approach the thyroid gland using an access further away. Ikeda et al. [8] performed a series of endoscopic thyroidectomy using the axilla approach with CO_2 insufflation. Higher satisfaction score together with higher pain scores were found in their group of patients underwent thyroidectomy by the axillary approach than those patients underwent video-assisted approach using small suprasternal incision [9]. Ohgami et al. [10] reported endoscopic thyroidectomy via the breast approach with low-pressure subcutaneous CO_2 insufflation. Three trocars are inserted into the breast and parasternal area. The vessels and parenchymal dissection are achieved by ultrasonic shear as well. This approach is also favored by surgeons in the mainland China because of a familial anatomical view to conventional surgery and the relatively shorter learning curve [11]. However, hypertrophic scars may develop in the parasternal port. Shimazu et al. [12] developed another technique by converting the parasternal region to axilla region on the tumor side to increase the viewing angle. This approach is named the axillo-bilateral-breast approach (ABBA).

Korean surgeons also put a lot of efforts in the development of endoscopic thyroidectomy via remote access. The most popular methods are the gasless transaxillary approach (GTA) [13] and the bilateral axillo-breast approach (BABA) [14] which will be illustrated later.

Besides, there are also reports on approach via a more remote access. These include the postauricular-areolar approach [15], the trans-areola single-incision approach [16], the transoral thyroidectomy [17] as well as the facelift thyroidectomy [18] using da Vinci surgical robotic system.

I am going to outline the two most common methods in the following paragraphs, namely the gasless transaxillary approach and bilateral axillo-breast approach.

Gasless Transaxillary Approach (GTA)

The gasless transaxillary approach was pioneered by Chung WY [13,19-26] from Yonsei University in year 2001. In his original version, a 3.5cm vertical incision is made at the axilla. Another 0.5cm skin incision is made near at the chest wall on ipsilateral side to the tumor. The subcutaneous flap is raised by sharp dissection. The working space is then maintained by the Chung's retractor without CO_2 insufflation. Surgery can be performed under a clear endoscopic view. The recurrent laryngeal nerve can be clearly identified. Robotic da Vinci Surgical System can be docked in after skin flap is developed and stabilized by the Chung's retractor [13,19,31]. A suction catheter is connected to the retractor to suck out the vapour and smoke in the operative field. In their later series, they are able to perform the surgery with a single vertical 5-6cm incision at axilla without the need for an additional chest port [21]. There are a number reports showing success in this approach for the management of benign thyroid lesions [13,19-21,31], Graves' disease [22] as well as early thyroid cancers [13,20,23-25,39]. Modified radical neck dissection can be performed in the same setting in patients with lateral neck lymph node metastasis [23]. The main criticism for this approach is the limited view and access for contralateral thyroid lobe as well as the contralateral recurrent laryngeal nerve. Since the anatomy is unfamiliar to most general surgeon, the reported learning curve is steep [25-26]. They suggest the learning curve for GTA is around 55-60 cases by endoscopic surgery and 35-40 cases by robotic surgery [25].

Bilateral Axillo-Breast Approach (BABA)

Another Korean surgeon, Youn YK [14,27-30] from the Seoul National University and Hospital, has developed another method using 4-port approach towards bilateral areolar and axilla, which is known as the bilateral axillo-breast approach (BABA). The subplatysmal flap is initially raised by injection of diluted epinephrine as "hydro-dissection". The plane is developed by blunt dissection of a vascular tunneler from the areola / axilla wound directly towards the thyroid cartilage. CO_2 insufflation can be maintained at 6-8mmHg to avoid patient having hypercapnia. The remaining flap dissection is mainly performed by ultrasonic dissector or diathermy hook under direct videoscopic guidance. After full visualization of recurrent laryngeal nerve and parathyroid glands, thyroidectomy is performed using Harmonic Scalpel. In case total thyroidectomy is contemplated, this can be performed using the same trocars. The specimen is put into a plastic bag and retrieved through the axilla port. After meticulous haemostasis, midline is closed with endo-suture. A suction drain is left in place. The skin wound is approximated with sutures and proper compression of the skin flap is applied postoperatively.

The main advantage of this approach is good exposure for both sides as well as a familiar anatomical view as in conventional open surgery. This main criticism for this approach is the blunt trauma in development of a wide flap which may cause paraesthesia over the anterior chest. Kim et al. [30] has shown that the change in sensation of the anterior chest can be recovered in 3 months after BABA thyroidectomy. Nevertheless, patients from western countries especially the United States are very reluctant to have the incisions placed over their breasts or areolae for endoscopic thyroidectomy.

DA Vinci Robotic Thyroidectomy

With the development of da Vinci Robotic Surgical System, surgeons can work in a narrow space with fine movement, dissection and suturing due to the dexterity of robotic arm. The three-dimensional magnified view may help the surgeons to overcome the limitations of endoscopic thyroidectomy.

Korean surgeons who developed endoscopic thyroidectomy also started their gasless transaxillary thyroidectomy and BABA thyroidectomy by using robot assistance in 2007 and 2008 and reported their works afterwards [20-30]. The robotic procedure is basically the same as the endoscopic thyroidectomy. By having robotic assistance, the learning curve may be shorten and more lymph nodes may be retrieved compared to endoscopic surgery as reported in a multicenter trial [25].

The gasless transaxillary robotic thyroidectomy technique is learnt and practiced by surgeons from the United States [32-35] and some European countries [36].

Role in Cancer Surgery

MIVAT procedure is shown to be having less postoperative pain and better aesthetic result. Furthermore, prospective studies also showed that MIVAT can be used for patients diagnosed to have small differentiated thyroid cancer (<2cm in size) with a small thyroid volume (<25ml) and without evidence of neck lymph node metastasis [37-38].

Korean surgeons have the greatest experiences of performing thyroid cancer surgery using robot assistance, either by GTA or BABA techniques [20-30]. Lee et al. [28] has compared the robotic BABA versus conventional surgery by propensity score matching. The surgical completeness of both procedures is not differed and so the author suggests that patients with small thyroid cancers who prefer scarless neck surgery can consider robotic BABA procedure. Another Korean surgeon Lee et al. [39] showed there is no difference on the number of central compartment lymph nodes, postoperative stimulated thyroglobulin level as well as the radioactive iodine uptake between robotic GTA and conventional open surgery.

Our Local Experience

We have started endoscopic thyroidectomies since 2009. Different approaches had been performed using including bilateral axillo-breast approach (BABA), breast approach as described by Ohgami [10] [Figure 2] as well as axillo-bilateral breast approach (ABBA) [Figure 3]. Majority of our cases of endoscopic thyroidectomy are using breast approach [40]. To overcome the narrow angle view from this approach, sometimes we can use a hook inserted through the patients' neck for retraction of sternocleidomastoid muscle [Figure 4].

In Hong Kong, there are only 6 robotic machines available at the moment. This limited the chances of surgeons being trained and exposed to robotic surgery. Cost is another issue that hindered the use of robotic surgery other than the most common indications like prostatectomy and total mesorectal excision of rectal tumors.

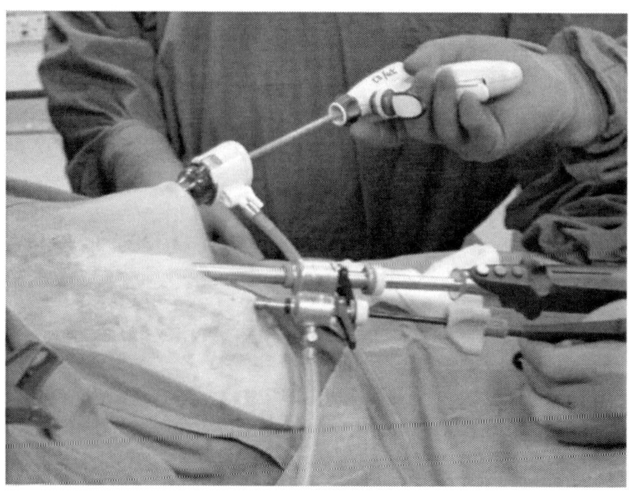

Figure 2. Endoscopic thyroidectomy using breast approach.

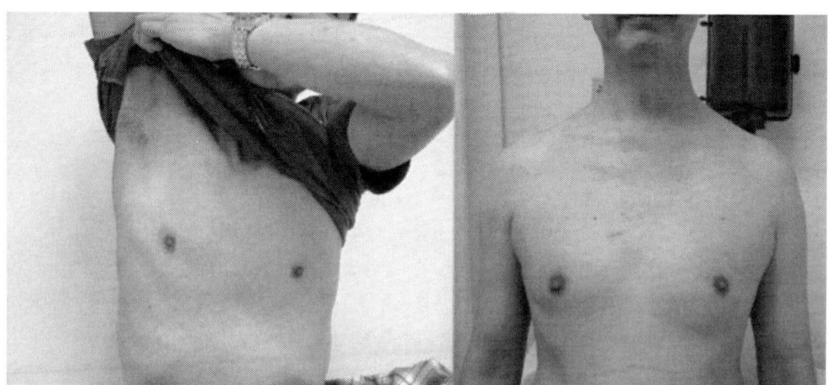

Figure 3. Male patients underwent endoscopy thyroidectomy by ABBA (*left side*) and breast approach (*right side*).

We are one of the surgical centers in Hong Kong that is practicing robotic thyroidectomy [41]. We perform BABA robotic thyroidectomy for the majority of our cases [Figure 5 & 6]. We have to ensure optimal patient position with application of protection foams before starting the procedure [Figure 7]. In the subplatysmal dissection, we use 'hydro-dissection' method as described in the BABA technique [14]. However, we try to keep the blunt dissection by tunneler to a minimum in order to decrease the chest wall bruises after surgery [Figure 8]. The flap can then be raised by Harmonic Scalpel.

Once the working space is enough for the docking, we dock the da Vinci robotic machine to continue the final step in the creation of the working space. A clear view can be obtained in robotic camera view. With a better depth perception and a clear magnified view, we think that important structures like recurrent laryngeal nerves and parathyroid glands can be identified in more details compared to endoscopic thyroidectomy.

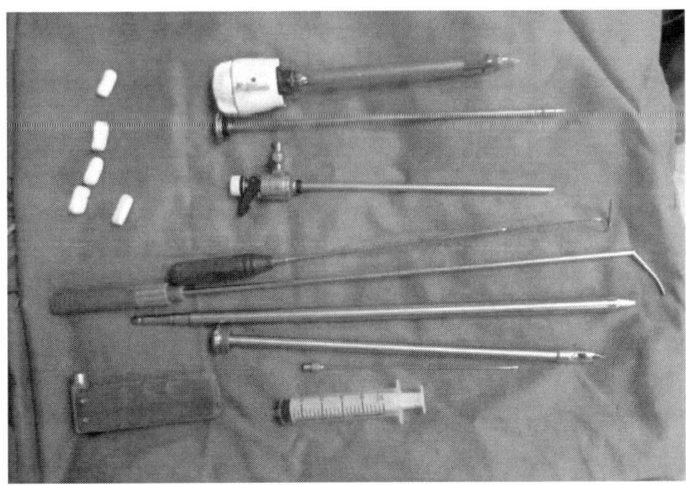

Figure 4. Instruments for endoscopic thyroidectomy (*list from above downwards*). a) Endo-peanut swab (upper left corner), b) Transparent 12mm long trocar, c) 5mm metal long trocar, d) Curve hook for retraction of sternocleidomastoid muscle (optional), e) 5mm thyroid dissector, f) Subcutaneous tunneler, g) Blunt tip needle for injection of diluted epinephrine, h) Handle for the subtaneous tunneler (lower left, corner), i) 20ml syringe.

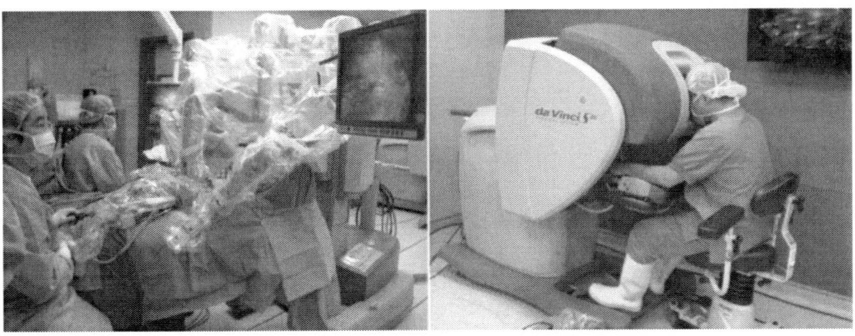

Figure 5. Robotic BABA procedure. *Left side:* Patient side. *Right side:* Console surgeon.

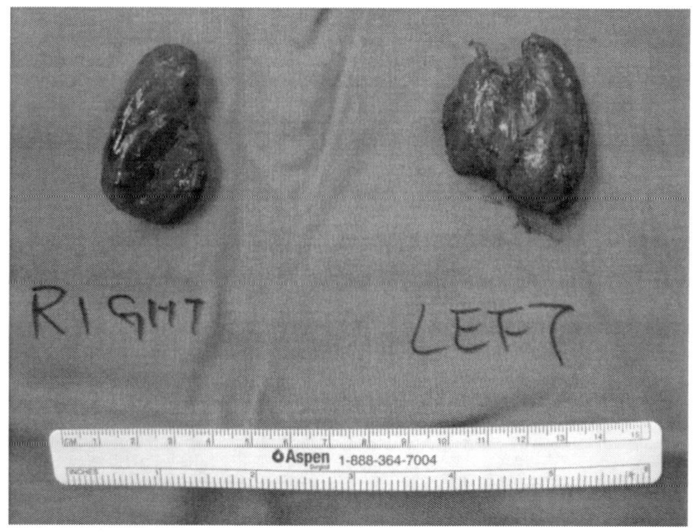

Figure 6. Surgical specimen for robotic BABA total thyroidectomy.

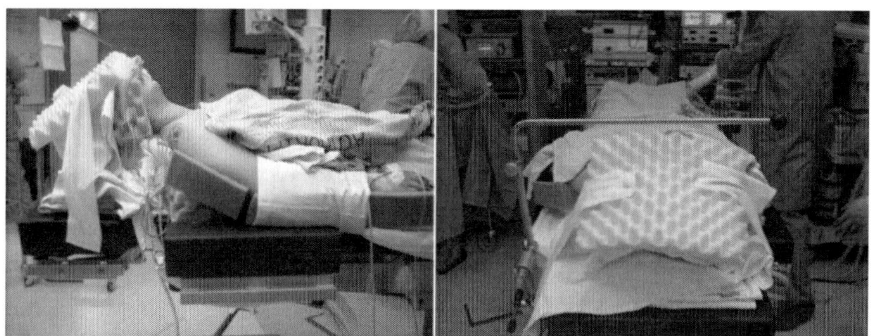

Figure 7. Patient's position for robotic BABA thyroidectomy.

Until 2013, we have completed more than 50 cases of robotic thyroidectomy using the BABA technique and a few cases of robotic gasless transaxillary thyroidectomy [Figure 9]. Indications and contraindications for robotic thyroidectomy are listed in Table 1. Our result of patients underwent endoscopic thyroidectomy via breast approach and robotic thyroidectomy using BABA technique during year 2010-2013 is shown. The patients' characteristics are shown in Table 2. Female predominance is noticed and older patients are found in the endoscopic group. Only one-fourth of our patients underwent total thyroidectomy. The hospital stay is longer for robotic surgery. The size of thyroid and size of tumor are similar for both groups [Table 3]. 16-19% of our cases are malignant on final histology and most of them are papillary microcarcinoma or papillary carcinoma. We have encountered more recurrent laryngeal nerve injuries in the endoscopic group, which are mainly happened during our early learning curve period [Table 4]. A possible reason is due to the heat transferred by hot surgical instruments like Harmonic Scalpel. Hypertrophic scars were found at the parasternal port site of two patients. One patient in robotic group developed haematoma in the neck postoperatively. Re-laparoscopy through the original working ports showed that the bleeding was originated from the camera port site. The bleeding was controlled by surgical sutures.

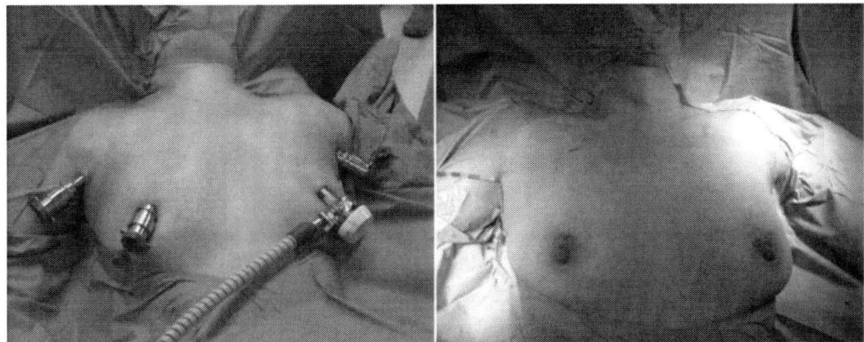

Figure 8. Robotic BABA thyroidectomy. *Left side:* Port placement. *Right side:* Immediate postoperative photo with drainage catheter on patient's right axilla.

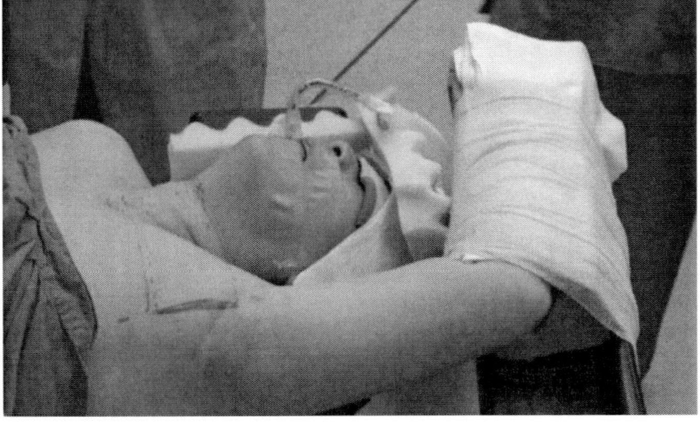

Figure 9. Patient's position for gasless robotic transaxillary thyroidectomy.

Table 1. Indications and contraindications for robotic thyroidectomy

Indications	Thyroid nodule <= 5cm size Papillary carcinoma < 2cm size Follicular lesion Follicular neoplasm Indeterminate thyroid nodules on cytology
Relative Contraindications	Posterior located tumor Graves' disease with relapse (under control) Tumor size > 5cm Lymph node metastasis in lateral neck Underlying chronic obstructive airway disease
Absolute Contraindications	Uncontrolled thyrotoxicosis Retrosternal goiter Thyroiditis Tumor invasion to recurrent laryngeal nerve, trachea, oesophagus and great vessels Patient's refusal to robotic surgery

Table 2. Patient's characteristics for endoscopic and robotic thyroidectomy in 2010-2013

	Endoscopic Breast approach (N=75)	**Robotic BABA (N=51)**	***p* Value**
Median Age of patients (years)*	52 (20 – 79)	43 (17-63)	**0.01**[a]
Sex			**0.026**[a]
male	10 (13%)	1 (2%)	
female	65 (87%)	50 (98%)	
Extension of resection			0.849[a]
Hemithyroidectomy	57 (76%)	38 (75%)	
Total thyriodectomy	18 (24%)	13 (25%)	
Length of postoperative hospital stay (days)*	1 (1-10)	2 (1-9)	**<0.01**[b]

* Median and range in parenthesis.

[a] Chi-square test.

[b] Mann-Whitney U test.

Bold signifies $p < 0.05$.

Table 3. Tumor characteristics and operative outcome of endoscopic and robotic thyroidectomy (2010-2013)

	Endoscopic Breast approach (N=75)	Robotic BABA (N=51)	*p* Value
Size of tumor (mm)*	23 (1-62)	20 (2-50)	0.365[b]
Size of gland (mm)*	53 (30-100)	54 (15-80)	0.556[b]
Specimen weight (g)*	24 (5-138)	21 (4-82)	0.06[b]
Operating time (mins)*	130 (55-382)	220 (85-600)	**<0.01[b]**
Blood loss (ml)*	3 (0-800)	20 (1-200)	**<0.01[b]**
Final Histology			0.154[a]
Benign	61 (81%)	43 (84%)	
Malignant	14 (19%)	8 (16%)	
Malignant Histology			0.400[a]
PTMC	8	3	
Papillary Carcinoma	4	4	
Follicular Carcinoma (minimally invasive)	2	1	

* Median and range in parenthesis.
[a] Chi-square test.
[b] Mann-Whitney U test.
Bold signifies $p < 0.05$.
PTMC – papillary microcarcinoma.

Table 4. Postoperative complications of endoscopic and robotic thyroidectomy (2010-2013)

	Endoscopic Breast approach (n=75)	Robotic BABA (n =51)
Open conversion	0	0
Complications		
Bleeding/haematoma	0	1 (re-exploration)
Transient RLN palsy	3	1
Permanent RLN palsy	3	0
Hypoparathyroidism	0	2
Hypertrophic scars	2	0

Discussion

As the beginning of this new procedure, many surgeons suggest to start off with small and benign lesions, followed by indeterminate lesion. The use of endoscopoic and robotic thyroidectomy is still controversial for malignant thyroid lesions although large scale series are reported by the Korean surgeons.

The excellent postoperative outcomes are usually seen in Korean series. Majority of these reports are coming from a single center, or even with single chief surgeons who operate on a large number of cases and become proficient in this procedure. Therefore, this is definitely difficult repeat such excellent results in low volume centers.

There is a report of case series of 100 cases from the United States [33]. However, there are also reports on serious complications which have never been happened in conventional thyroidectomy like persistent chest wall numbness, brachial plexus injury and oesophageal perforation [42]. The Food and Drug Administration in the United States has revoked the approval on the use of robot for thyroidectomy in October 2011 [43]. Experience endocrine surgeons who introduced robot-assisted GTA in the United States indeed stop using this technique [43-46]. Lino D has studied the patient's attitude towards GTA in Greece [47]. It was found that only 11.6% of the patients in the study group prefer to have thyroidectomy by the robotic transaxillary method. The underlying reasons given include various perceived disadvantages of the robotic procedure (increase pain, longer operative time, and higher cost).

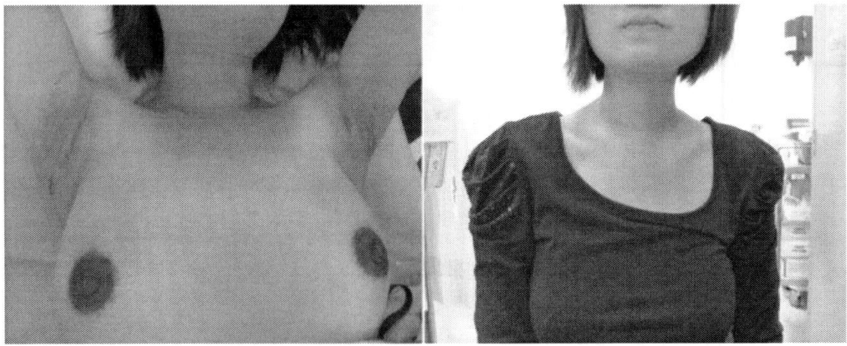

Figure 10. Patient's postoperative photo one week after robotic BABA thyroidectomy.

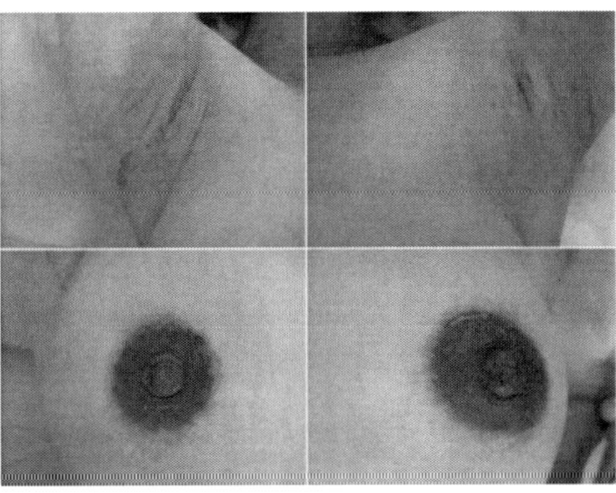

Figure 11. Magnified view of patient in Figure 10 after robotic BABA thyroidectomy.

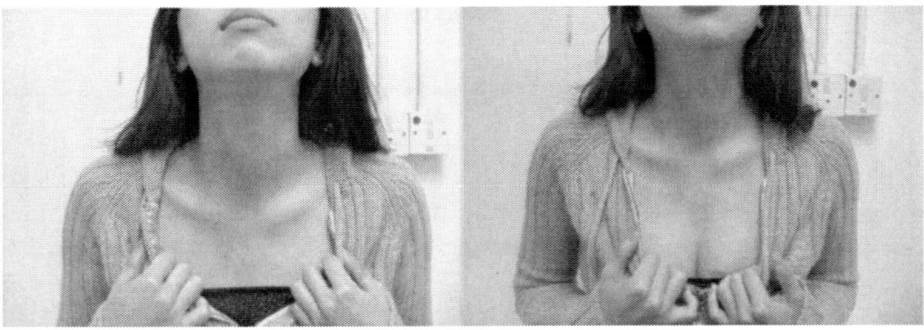

Figure 12. Postoperative photo three months after endoscopoic thyroidectomy using breast approach. The parasternal wound (*left side*) can be completely covered by patient's clothes.

In the development of minimally invasive surgical procedures, the common quoted benefits are shorter operating time, less postoperative pain, shorter hospital stay, early recovery and comparable result to open surgery for oncological clearance. However, this is not the case for endoscopic or robotic thyroid surgeries. With an additional tunnel or skin flap as access wound, the access trauma towards the patients may cause pain. Some of the patients may also complain of paraesthesia over the anterior chest wall. The additional working tunnel will also increase a potential space of seroma formation. Therefore we put in a suction drain liberally after endoscopic thyroidectomy and robotic thyroidectomy.

Another important drawback of robotic thyroidectomy is the cost of surgery. The cost of robotic surgery is the highest, followed by endoscopic surgery. Conventional open thyroidectomy, the gold standard, is also having the lowest cost [48,49]. Decreasing the operating time will reduce the cost differences theoretically. From a cost analysis in the United States, endoscopic GTA needs to be decreased to 111 minutes and robotic GTA needs to be decreased 68 minutes in order to make the cost equivalent to conventional surgery [49]. This is not feasible especially in low volume surgical centers.

A recently published systemic review [50] showed that robotic thyroidectomy has not demonstrated superiority in comparison with conventional open surgery in terms of operating time, hospital stay and temporary recurrent laryngeal nerve palsy rates. Expensive instruments, increasing number of consumables, extra training in surgical staff as well as theatre nurses are required. The most significant benefit is the good cosmetic outcome with the wound hidden in the axilla or around the areola [Figure 10-12].

Conclusion

At the present moment, conventional surgery is still the gold standard for thyroid surgery. Endoscopic and robotic thyroidectomies are not widely practiced in the world. These procedures are still preferred to be done in high volume surgical centers. Although good and favorable cosmetic outcome can be achieved in the group of carefully selected patients, we should have a throughout discussion with our patients about the pros and cons of these procedures before proceeding to surgery.

References

[1] Gagner, M. Endoscopic subtotal parathyroidectomy in patients with primary hyperparathyroidism. *Br J Surg.*, 1996, 83(6), 875.

[2] Hüscher, CS; Chiodini, S; Napolitano, C; Recher, A. Endoscopic right thyroid lobectomy. *Surg Endosc.*, 1997, 11(8), 877.

[3] Miccoli, P; Berti, P; Conte, M; Bendinelli, C; Marcocci, C. Minimally invasive surgery for small thyroid nodules: preliminary report. *J Endocrinol Invest.*, 1999, 22(11), 849-851.

[4] Miccoli, P; Berti, P; Raffelli, M; Materazzi, G; Baldacci, S; Rossi, G. Comparison between minimally invasive video-assisted thyroidectomy and conventional thyroidectomy: a prospective randomized study. *Surgery.*, 2001, 130(6), 1039-1043.

[5] Inabnet, WB; Jacob, PB; Gagner, M. Minimally invasive endoscopic thyroidectomy by a cervical approach: early vessel ligation decreases duration of surgery. *Surg Endosc.*, 2003, 17(11), 1808-1811.

[6] Shimizu, K; Arika, S; Jasmi, AY; Kitamura, Y; Kitagawa, W; Akasu, H; Tanaka, S. Video-assisted neck surgery: endoscopic resection of thyroid tumors with a minimal neck wound. *J Am Coll Surg.*, 1999, 188 (6), 697-703.

[7] Shimizu, K; Tanaka, S. Asian perspective on endoscopic thyroidectomy – a review of 193 cases. *Asian J Surg.*, 2003, 26(2), 92-100.

[8] Ikeda, Y; Takami, H; Sasaki, Y; Kan, S; Niimi, M. Endoscopic neck surgery by the axillary approach. *J Am Coll Surg.*, 2000, 191(3), 336-340.

[9] Ikeda, Y; Takami, H; Sasaki, Y; Takayama, JI; Kurihara, H. Are there significant benefits of minimally invasive endoscopic thyroidectomy. *World J Surg.*, 2004, 28(11), 1075-1078.

[10] Ohgami, M; Ishii, S; Arisawa, Y; Ohmori, T; Noga, K; Furukawa, T; Kitajima, M. Scarless endoscopic thyroidectomy: breast approach for better cosmesis. *Surg Laparosc Endosc.*, 2000, 10(1), 1-4.

[11] Cao, F; Jin, K; Cui, B; Xie, B. Learning curve for endoscopic thyroidectomy: a single teaching hospital study. *Onco Target Ther.*, 2013, 6, 47-52.

[12] Shimazu, K; Shiba, E; Tamaki, Y; Takiguchi, S; Taniguchi, E; Ohashi, S; Noguchi, S. Endoscopic thyroid surgery through the axillo-bilateral-breast approach. *Surg Laparosc Endosc Percut Tech.*, 2003, 13(3), 196-201.

[13] Yoon, JH; Park, CH; Chung, WY. Gasless endoscopic thyroidectomy via an axillary approach: report of 30 cases. *Surg Laparosc Endosc Percut Tech.*, 2006, 16(4), 226-231.

[14] Choe, JH; Kim, SW; Chung, KW; Park, SK; Han, W; Noh, DY; Oh, SK; Youn, YK. Endoscopic thyroidectomy using a new bilateral axillo-breast approach. *World J Surg.*, 2007, 31(3), 601-606.

[15] Kim, SJ; Lee, KE; Lee, J; Koo, DH; Youn, YK; Oh, SK. Postauricular and axillary approach endoscopic thyroidectomy with the da vinci robotic system. *Int J Med Robot Comp Assist Surg.*, 2011, 7, 40.

[16] Youben, F; Bomin, G; Bo, W; Jie, K; Fan, Y; Wencai, Q; Yuyao, H; Qi, Z. Trans-areola single-incision endoscopic thyroidectomy. *Surg Laparosc Endosc Percut Tech.*, 2011, 21(4), e192-e196.

[17] Nakajo, A; Arima, H; Hirata, M; Mizoguchi, T; Kijima, Y; Mori, S; Ishigami, S; Ueno, S; Yoshinaka, H; Natsugoe, S. Trans-oral video-

assisted neck surgery (TOVANS). A new transoral technique of endoscopic thyroidectomy with gasless premandible approach. *Surg Endosc.*, 2013, 27(4), 1105-1110.

[18] Terris, DJ; Singer, MC; Seybt, MW. Robotic facelift thyroidectomy: patient selection and technical consideration. *Surg Laparosc Endosc Percut Tech.*, 2011, 21(4), 237-242.

[19] Kang, SW; Jeong, JJ; Yun, JS; Sung, TV; Lee, SC; Lee, YS; Nam, KH; Chang, HS., Chung, WY; Park, CS. Gasless endoscopic thyroidectomy using trans-axillary approach; surgical outcome of 581 patients. *Endocr J.*, 2009, 56(3), 361-369.

[20] Kang, SW; Jeong, JJ; Nam, KH; Chang, HS; Chung, WY; Park, CS. Robot-assisted endoscopic thyroidectomy for thyroid malignancies using a gasless transaxillary approach. *J Am Coll Surg.*, 2009, 209(2), e1-e7.

[21] Ryu, HR; Kang, SW; Lee, SH; Rhee, KY; Jeong, JJ; Nam, KH; Chung, WY; Park, CS. Feasibility and safety of a new robotic thyroidectomy through a gasless, transaxillary single-incision approach. *J Am Coll Surg.*, 2010, 211(3), e13-e19.

[22] Park, JH; Lee, CR; Park, S; Jeong, JS; Kang, SW; Jeong, JJ; Nam, KH; Chung, WY; Park, CS. Initial experience with robotic gasless transaxillary thyroidectomy for the management of Graves' disease, comparison of conventional open versus robotic thyroidectomy. *Surg Laparosc Endosc Percutan Tech.*, 2013, 23(5), e173-e177.

[23] Kang, SW; Lee, SH; Park, JH; Jeong, JS; Park, S; Lee, CR; Jeong, JJ; Nam, KH; Chung, WY; Park, CS. A comparative study of the surgical outcomes of robotic and conventional open modified radical neck dissection for papillary thyroid carcinoma with lateral neck node metastasis. *Surg Endosc.*, 2012, 26(11), 3251-3257.

[24] Lee, J; Yun, JH; Nam, KH; Soh, EY; Chung, WY. The learning curve for robotic thyroidectomy: a multicenter study. *Ann Surg Oncol.*, 2011, 18(1), 226-232.

[25] Lee, J; Yun, JH; Choi, UJ; Kang, SW; Jeong, JJ; Chung, WY. Robotic versus endoscopic thyroidectomy for thyroid cancers: a multi-institutional analysis of early postoperative outcomes and surgical learning curves. *J Oncol.*, 2012, 2012, 734541.

[26] Lee, J; Lee, JH; Nah, KY; Soh, EY; Chung, WY. Comparison of endoscopic and robotic thyroidectomy. *Ann Surg Oncol.*, 2011, 18(5), 1439-1446.

[27] Lee, KE; Rao, J; Youn, YK. Endoscopic thyroidectomy with the da vinci robotic system using the bilateral axillary breast approach (BABA) technique. *Surg Laparosc Endosc Percutan Tech.*, 2009, 19(3), e71-e75.

[28] Lee, KE; Koo, DH; Im, HJ; Park, SK; Choi, JY; Paeng, JC; Chung, JK; Oh, SK; Youn, YK. Surgical completeness of bilateral axillo-breast approach robotic thyroidectomy: comparison with conventional open thyroidectomy after propensity score matching. *Surgery*, 2011, 150(6), 1266-1274.

[29] Lee, KE; Koo, DH; Kim, SJ; Lee, J; Park, KS; Oh, SK; Youn, YK. Outcomes of 109 patients with papillary thyroid carcinoma who underwent robotic total thyroidectomy with central node dissection via the bilateral axillo-breast approach. *Surgery*, 2010, 148(6), 1207-1213.

[30] Kim, SJ; Lee, KE; Myong, JP; Koo, DH; Lee, J; Youn, YK. Prospective study of sensation in anterior chest areas before and after a bilateral axillo-breast approach for endoscopic / robotic thyroid surgery. *World J Surg.*, 2013, 37(5), 1147-1153.

[31] Giannopoulos, G; Kang, SW; Jeong, JJ; Nam, KH; Chung, WY. Robotic thyroidectomy for benign thyroid diseases: a stepwise strategy to the adoption of robotic thyroidectomy (gasless, transaxillary approach). *Surg Laparosc Endosc Percut Tech.*, 2013(3), 23, 312-315.

[32] Kuppersmith, RB, Holsinger, FC. Robotic thyroid surgery: an initial experience with North American patients. *Laryngoscope*, 2011, 121(3), 521-526.

[33] Kandil, EH; Noureldine, SI; Yao, L; Slakey, D. Robotic transaxillary thyroidectomy: an examination of the first one hundred cases. *J Am Coll Surg.*, 2012, 214(4), 558-566.

[34] Lin, HS; Folbe, AJ; Carron, MA; Zuliani; Chen, W; Yoo, GH; Mathog, RH. Single-incision transaxillary robotic thyroidectomy: challenges and limitations in a North American population. *Otolaryngol Head Neck Surg.*, 2012, 147(6), 1041-1046.

[35] Landry, CS; Grubbs; EG; Warneke, CL; Ormond, M; Chua, C; Lee, JE; Perrier, ND. Robot-assisted transaxillary thyroid surgery in the United States: is it comparable to open thyroid lobectomy? *Ann Surg Oncol.*, 2012, 19(4), 1269-1274.

[36] Axente, DD; Silaghi, H; Silaghi, CA; Major, ZZ; Micu, CM; Constantea, NA. Operative outcomes of robot-assisted transaxillary thyroid surgery for benign thyroid disease: early experience in 50 patients. *Langenbecks Arch Surg.*, 2013, 398(6), 887-894.

[37] Paolo, DR; Lucia, S; Paola, P; Simona, P; Francesca, AM; Macro, F; Mario, S. Minimally invasive video-assisted thyroidectomy in differentiated thyroid cancer: a 1-year follow up. *Surg Laparosc Endosc Percut Tech.*, 2009, 19(4), 290-292.

[38] Pisanu, A; Podda, M; Reccia, I; Porceddu, G; Uccheddu, A. Systematic review with meta-analysis of prospective randomized trials comparing minimally invasive video-assisted thyroidectomy (MIVAT) and conventional thyroidectomy. *Langenbecks Arch Surg.*, 2013, 398(8), 1057-1068.

[39] Lee, S; Lee, CR; Lee, SC; Park, S; Kim, HY; Son, H; Kang, SW; Jeong, JJ; Nam, KH; Chung, WY; Park, CS; Cho, A. Surgical completeness of robotic thyroidectomy: a prospective comparison with conventional open thyroidectomy in papillary thyroid carcinoma patients. *Surg Endosc.*, 2014, 28(4), 1068-1075.

[40] Yau, KK; Tsui, DK; Li, MK. Endoscopic thyroidectomy. *Surg Practice.*, 2011, 15(1), 27-28.

[41] Tsui, DK; Yau, KK; Tang, CN. Robotic thyroidectomy using bilateral axillo-breast approach. *Surg Practice*, 2013, 17(3), 127-128.

[42] Patel, D; Kebebew, E. Pros and cons of robotic transaxillary thyroidectomy. *Thyroid*, 2012, 22(10), 984-985.

[43] Inabnet, WB, III. Robotic thyroidectomy: must we drive a luxury sedan to arrive at our destination safely? *Thyroid*, 2012, 22(10), 988-990.

[44] Linos, D. Less is more: the example of minimally invasive thyroidectomy. *JAMA Surgery*, 2013, 148(9), 808-809.

[45] Perrier, ND. Why I have abandoned robot-assisted transaxillary thyroid surgery. *Surgery*, 2012, 152(6), 1025-1026

[46] Duh, QY. Robot-assisted endoscopic thyroidectomy: has the time come to abandon neck incisions? *Ann Surg*, 2011, 253(6), 1067-1068.

[47] Linos, D; Kiriakopoulos, A; Petralias, A. Patient attitudes toward transaxillary robot-assisted thyroidectomy. *World J Surg.*, 2013, 37(8), 1959-1965.

[48] Broome, JT; Pomeroy, S; Solorzano, CC. Expense of robotic thyroidectomy – a cost analysis at a single institution. *Arch Surg.*, 2012, 147(12), 1102-1106.

[49] Cabot, JC; Lee, CR; Brunaud, L; Kleiman, A; Chung, WY; Fahey, TJ; Zarnegar, R. Robotic and endoscopic transaxillary thyroidectomies may be cost prohibitive when compared to standard cervical thyroidectomy: a cost analysis. *Surgery*, 2012, 152(6), 1016-1024.

[50] Lang, BH; Wong, CK; Tsang, JS; Wong, KP; Wan, KY. A systemic review and meta-analysis comparing surgically-related complications between robotic-assisted thryoidectomy and conventional open thyroidectomy. *Ann Surg Oncol*, 2014, 21(3), 850-861.

In: Thyroidectomy
Editor: Kimberly Rodolfo
ISBN: 978-1-63321-440-8

Chapter 8

Thyroid Pathology: Our Experience

José Luis D'Addino and Maria Mercedes Pigni
Head and Neck Surgery.Vicente Lopez Public Hospital.
Buenos Aires, Argentina
Vicente Lopez Public Hospital, Adolfo Alsina, Florida,
Vicente López, Buenos Aires, Argentina

Abstract

A review of 814 thyroid surgery performed in a Public Hospital at Buenos Aires is presented in order to compare our statistic with international reports. We compare sex, age, pathology, histological type, surgical procedures, complications and associated treatment to surgery in malignant tumors.

Keyword: Thyroid Pathology

Introduction

This Chapter is about a review of our Head and Neck Section's statistic of general thyroid pathology that we had operated at Vicente Lopez Public Hospital, between January 2004 and 2010.

The total of patients were 814. The malignant pathology represented 229 cases. The statistic study is made considering: age, sex, histologicaltype, type of surgery, treatment with iodine 131 and the negativization in the scintigraphy scan and the assay of thyroglobulin. We compare complications and surgical procedures.

Materials and Methods

We have analyzed 814 patients. All of them underwent to a surgical procedure with benign or malignant pathology diagnosed. Statistical differences were calculated for sex and pathology and the mean age. It is used: media, average, percentage, statistical test of sensitivity.

Histological differences in malignant pathologies were considered: aggressively, extrathyroideal invasion, local or distance metastases.

All of the histological samples were studied with Hematoxylin and eosin; and when resulted necessary, we used immunohistochemistry marking.

We mention uncommon malignant cases with unusual presentation operated in our Service.

All patients were studied by laboratory, ultrasound, CT scan, scintigraphy scan, and fine needle aspiration. Eventually we performed a MRI or PET scan.

Surgeries have been performed by the same equipment and the surgical procedures were: Benign pathology; total or subtotal thyroidectomy by cervicotomy, average section (6 cm). A "minicervicotomy" (3 cm) was performed if a single node is smaller than 1 x 1 cm and the patient had a thin neck. Referring to Malignant pathology; we always do total thyroidectomy by typical cervicotomy and if it is necessary, we enlarge the sectionl aterally in order to perform neck dissection. The internment's average staying was 24 hours.

The postoperative outcomes and complications are explained comparing to other authors.

Results

Total of patients operated because of thyroid pathology: 814 with a minimum age of 18 and maximum of 82, media: 50 years old. Total of surgeries were separated in 585 benign and 229 malignant. Considering the sex, 559 were female (95,5%) and 26 were male (4,48%) in relation to benign pathology(Figure 1). There is a big predominance of benign pathology in female but this predominance changes in malignant pathology. With a total of 229 malignant cases, 84,3%, 192 were female and 15,7%, 37 were male. This difference is statistical significantly ($P<0,01$) (Figure 2).

Benign Thyroid Pathology: the total of 585 patients operated are distributed as follows; Multinodular goiter 202 cases, (34,5%), 191 female and 11 male. Follicular adenoma in one solitary node 180 cases, (30,7%), 172 female and 18 male. In one case, we observed a Follicular adenoma papillary variant. Patients with hyperthyroidism derived for surgery because of no response with medical treatment (19,6%), 115 cases, 113 female and 2 male. Hashimoto Thyroiditis with nodes, 71 cases, (12,1%), 66 female and 5 male.

The rest of the benign pathology was: Hurtle adenoma in one node 10 cases, Oncocitic adenoma 4 cases, Quervain Thyroiditis 3, all of them female(Figure 3).

Malignant Thyroid Pathology: the total number of cases in this pathology was 229. The Papillary carcinoma represented the 74 %of all the malignant cases. In this case we are talking about 167 patients. Considering the papillary carcinoma, the classic type was the most common with 118 patients, (70%), 99 female and 19 male. Secondly we observed the Multicentric papillary carcinoma, 25 cases representing 14,9%, 19 female and 6 male. In this mentioned group, 90% had lymphatic metastases discovered at the operating room, all of them located at the "Recurrent area", level VI. Because of this reason, our election procedure in papillary carcinoma is total thyroidectomy regardless of tumor stage. Third place was the papillary carcinoma, follicular variant, 10 cases, 8 female and 2 male. In fourth place we observed the Papillary carcinoma with extrathyroide alinvation, 9 cases, all female. In this histological type we had 2 cases that resulted Tall cells. It also mentioned 4 cases of Squamous papillary carcinoma and 1 Diffuse sclerosing variant of the papillary type. 85 % of Papillary carcinoma was developed on a Hashimoto thyroiditis.

The following histological type in frequency was the Follicular carcinoma, 36 cases, (15,72 %), 30 female and 6 male.

The next malignant type was the Anaplastic carcinoma, 9 cases, (3,9%), 6 female and 3 male. Rare tumors were: Medullary carcinoma, 8 cases, (4%), 7 female, 1 male. Thyroid Lymphoma 3 cases, Squamous carcinoma 2 cases, Epithelioid Angiosarcoma 1 case, Mucoepidermoid carcinoma 1 case and 1 Plasmocitoma (Figure 4).

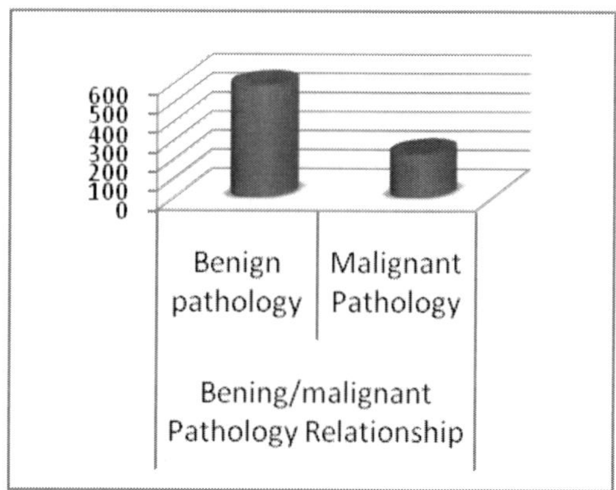

Figure 1. Pathology relationship.

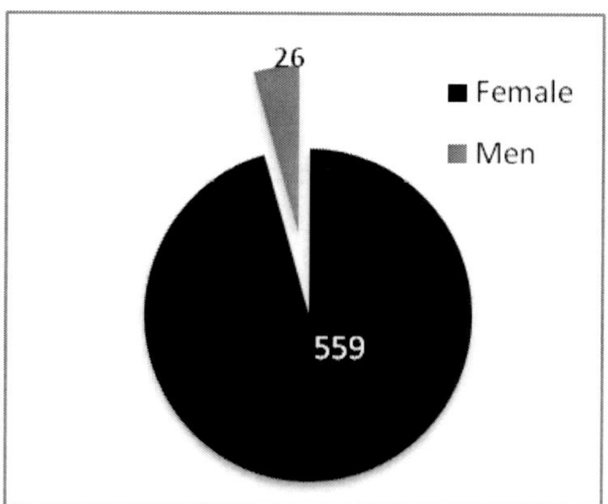

Figure 2. Sex relationship.

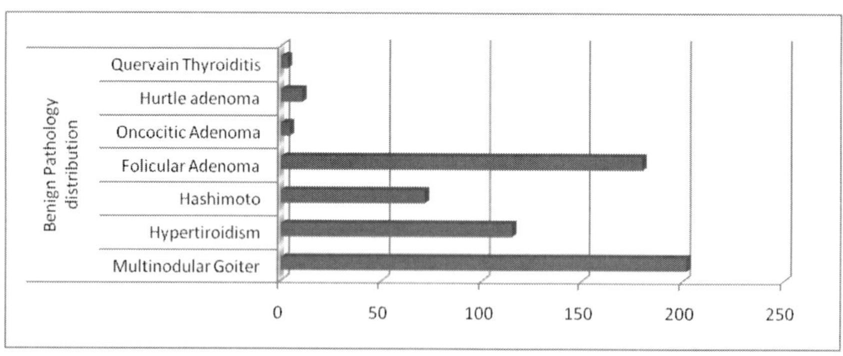

Figure 3. Benign pathology distribution.

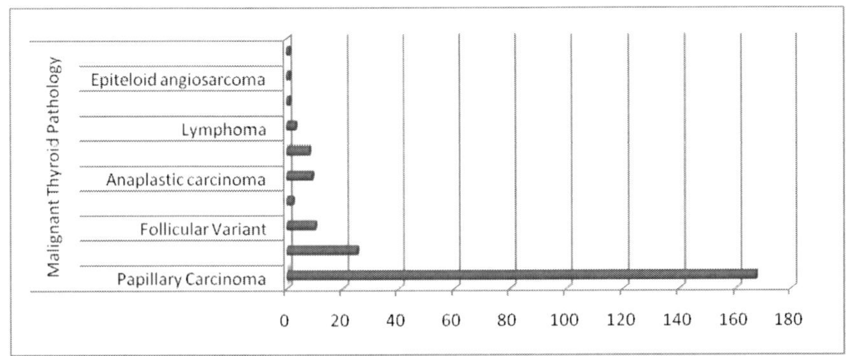

Figure 4. Malignant pathology distribution.

Thyroid metastases due to second carcinoma: 2 cases, one Clear cell carcinoma of the kidney operated 23 years earlier. The other case was one metastases of Endometrial carcinoma that appeared two years later.

Cervical Lymph node metastases: total 56 cases, 2 patients were because of Medullary carcinoma, the rest were in Papillary carcinoma type. In 1 woman we observed cystic metastases in a cervical lymph node, level V, with a size of 8 x 8 cm.

Intraoperative Frozen section histology: resulted positive in 80% but we obtained a false negative in 15 % of the cases that finally informed carcinoma. In 5% of the intra operative samples, the diagnosis was false positive for carcinoma and the deferred study was benign.

Post operative complication: in our series we registered 7 suffocating hematoma with one death, all of the cases related with hyperthyroidism. Recurrent palsy 12 cases (1,47% all in one nerve), 10 cases (1,1%) were only temporally with total recovery between 1 and 5 months; average: 3 months. Permanent paralysis of one nerve, 2 cases (0,2%), one due to recurrence of Basedow disease, in the second surgery and the other case due to extrathyroideal infiltration of Anaplastic carcinoma. We decided 10 tracheostomies in 5 Carcinomas, all the Anaplastic and Papillary carcinoma with extrathyroideal infiltration. In 5 opportunities the tracheostomy was made after a postoperative suffocating hematoma. One of these patients died because of acute respiratory depression, a woman with a Graves disease, hypertension and chronic obstructive pulmonary disease. The rest were decannulated between 1 and 2 months without any complication.

Hipoparathyroidism was reported in 20 cases (2,4%) temporally and in 2 cases (0,2%) definitive, these two patient were underwent to a total thyroidectomy with neck dissection and post operative dose of I^{131} and external radiotherapy because of malignant tumors.

No other complication related with the surgical procedure were found.

Scintigraphic screening post total thyroidectomy: it is frequent that oncologic patients after a total thyroidectomy have positive screening in scintigrahic scan with I^{131} especially in the surgical lodge. We had to re-operate patients in 8 cases and we found only 2 cases with neoplastic recurrence. The histology of the rest resulted fibrosis. The extracted volume average was 2 x 2 cm.

I^{131}Treatment: thyroid tumors are treated with Iodine after a total thyroidectomy using ablative dose. The most common is 100 mCi. Sometimes it is needed a second or a third dose of iodine. In our series, 70 % of the cases achieved negativization of the scintigraphic screening with one postoperative dose. 15 % needed 2 applications, 10 % received a third dose. 5 % required more than 3 doses.

Other treatments associated with thyroidectomy and I^{131}: in the Anaplastic carcinomas and the extrathyroideal infiltration carcinomas we used external radiotherapy in the cervical lodge and laterocervical areas. The average was 5.500 cGy. In one case we underwent a gastrostomy for feeding.

Mortality: 24 patients died, one female (0,17 %) because of a benign pathology, a suffocating hematoma which developed an acute respiratory depression. The other 23 cases (10,04 %) were related with malignant pathology in advanced stages.

Survival of carcinomas: the patients with classic papillary carcinoma, 118 cases recorded 98% of survival in 5 years. Considering all the Papillary types, the survival is 72 % in 5 years. The Follicular carcinoma had a survival of 100% and the Anaplastic carcinoma only 12 %. All the rare tumors founded, died before 5 years.

Discussion

According with international series, the nodular goiter has a prevalence of 2,5 % in the population and 7% predominates in female, specially in location with iodine deficiency. 5 to 15 % of the patients derived for surgery because of nodular goiter were carcinomas [1]. In our experience, 93% of the patients were female with a relation of 13/1 female/male. The average age was 46, 3 years old. 29,9 % had familiar heritage of thyroid disease, one patient had history of multiple endocrine disease. The benign pathology was the most frequent according with the international literature, in our chapter, 202 were benign pathology.

The follicular adenoma is frequent (30,7% in our series) but the papillary variant is uncommon, some authors mentioned that may exist papillary or pseudopapillary structures that may produce a confusion with the papillary carcinoma. The careful study of the specimen is important in order to avoid over diagnosis of papillary carcinoma. [2]

We have a higher casuistic than others in hyperthyroidism, represented in our study 19,6% of the benign pathology, the literature the frequency is 5%. This could be explained because of the low response to oral anti thyroid treatment in our population or incomplete treatment due to socioeconomic factors. In many places, the surgery is indicated when there are: failures with iodine treatment, goiter size, nodular goiter, anti thyroid allergy or drug intolerance, leucopenia, discontinue the oral therapy. We prefer the surgery as an initial treatment due to the economic factors in a Public Hospital and we have the possibility to make histological study of the gland.

The hyperthyroid crisis has an incidence of 10 % and the mortality rise to 20 %. This is the reason why all patients are blocked with high doses of oral Iodine, Lugol™(*Wolff-Chaikoff* effect) prior to the surgery. The recurrence with Iodine treatment is 5 to 28 %. In our experience, all the cases were operated, the recurrence were 2 women (1,7 %). Both with Basedow disease. Foreign Authors observed 1 to 33 % of recurrence when the residual post operative gland is more than 10 gr.(3)

With relation to malignant pathology, the Papillary carcinoma as a lonely node represented 70 %, similar with 80% reported in the international literature. Follicular carcinoma 15 % and Anaplastic 2 %. [2, 4]

Thyroid carcinoma is the 5th tumor in women, following the cancer breast, skin, uterus and colon. Risk factors in this pathology are the irradiation, heritage, diet, goiter, thyroiditis, estrogen. [5, 6, 7, 8, 9] The insulin resistance is now consider as another risk factor because of the association with the metabolic syndrome. [8, 10] In the Literature was described that the insulin resistance increase the thyroid gland and may develop nodules. Thyroid cells are sensitive to insulin and growth factors (IGF) I and II and TSH. TSH hormone is the most important factor in growth and follicular cells differentiation. [14, 15, 16, 17] This differentiation is associated with important changes in the expression of TSH and IGF receptors. [11, 12, 13]

Rezzonico J and col [18, 19] reported an increase of insulin resistance in patients with papillary carcinoma however these papillary carcinomas would be less aggressive.

The mortality has declined in the last three decades 50 %, the average mortality age is 73 years old. The Papillary carcinoma has increase the incidence and declined the mortality in women; in men it is observed an increase of mortality, especially over 50 years old and worst in advanced stages. 5 year survival in USA is 96,7%, considering stages, located disease 99,7%, local infiltration 96,9 % with cervical metastases 56 %. [6] 20 % of the Papillary carcinomas are multicenter from the beginning and 10% have local infiltration.

Some patients have high risk of local recurrence 5 to 20 % and may be related with incomplete treatment, tumor aggressiveness, and age. The most frequent localization are; the surgical lodge, lymphatic nodes and later distant metastases in lung and bones (10-15 %). [10] The recurrence is higher for the Tall cells Papillary carcinoma in youth under 16 years old and older than 45. The same situation occurs in the Diffuse Sclerosing type and in tumors with size bigger than 40 mm with extra thyroid infiltration. This is the reason why we underwent total thyroidectomy in all cases; this procedure allows us to complete a better follow up with Thyroglobulin, based on a negative scintigraphic screening.

Tall cells variant, described by Hawk and Hazard in 1976 [20] are more aggressive than classic Papillary carcinoma, in our experience, 2 cases, had tumors bigger than 5 cm with cervical metastases at the first visit to the Hospital. Both died in 3 years of follow up.

There are tumors that may have metastases with cystic transformation. The Papillary and the Epidermoid carcinoma are the most frequent in young people.(21) We operated 2 women that consulted at first because of laterocervical cyst. The histological study revealed Papillary carcinoma metastases with cystic transformation. There is less common clinical presentation such as solitary metastases, parapharyngeal mass. The occult carcinoma has a presentation of 15 %. [7, 8]

Diffuse sclerosing variant of the papillary type is rare, there are no statistics differences between sexes. In our review we have operated a man who consulted by cervical metastases mass. This type is associated with a mutation of the RET gen. The presentation is 2% in children and 10 % in adults. According with others authors, this tumor has a higher tendency to local infiltration and metastases. [22, 23, 24] Although it is more aggressive, the survival average is 93% in 10 years of follow up. [25, 26, 27] In our case, we needed 4 doses of Iodine^{131} (post total thyroidectomy associated with bilateral neck dissection) to obtain negativization of the scintigraphy scan and thyroglobulin.

Other uncommon type of thyroid tumor is the Squamous carcinoma variant of the papillary type. The most usual presentation is with a cervical mass. We underwent total thyroidectomy with neck dissection in 4 cases. Was initially observed that there was local tissue infiltration. All of them died before 5 years. [26] It is unknown its origin but seems to be an intense relation between cellular metaplasia (irradiation) and Hashimoto Thyroiditis.

Mucoepidermoid carcinoma of thyroid, was described by Chan in 1991. [27] We could find 35 cases in the International Literature, our case was the first in Argentina. The histogenesis of the variant sclerosing with eosinophylia mucoepidermoid carcinoma is related to a remnant of the last branchial body nevertheless some authors think that it could be developed by follicular cells directly. The patient we treated had a tumor of 4 x 4 cm without metastases. After a total thyroidectomy, we prescribed one ablative dose of iodine. He is actually free of disease. [28, 29]

Epithelioid Angiosarcoma was known formerly as hemangioendothelima and appeared especially in "alpine people". Rapidly metastasizing. Our case, a 66 years old man from Paraguay started symptoms with bone metastases (clavicle).

A total thyroidectomy with bilateral neck dissection a bone resection was performed. He died in 2 years. [30]

Metastases in thyroid gland is not frequent, our cases, a male and a woman had at the beginning local extra thyroid infiltration and lymph node metastases. One case was a renal tumor that was operated 23 years earlier and the other was a metastatic endometrial carcinoma operated 2 years earlier. Both are death.

The incidence of metastases found in autopsies was reported as 1-25 % in patient without a known primary and 24 % in patients with malignant primary. Mayo Clinic reported 43 patients with metastases in thyroid, the renal was the most common (33%) and the average time to appearance of metastases was 106 months. [31]

As postoperative complications we had 10 temporally recurrent nerve palsy, (1,2%) and 20 temporally hypoparathyroidism (2,4%). International Literature reported (3% and 2,6 %). 4 patients, 2 cases with Definitive nerve palsy and 2 definitive hypoparathyroidism (0,2 % in each case). Others Authors reported (1,9 and 0,2%). [32]

We registered 7 suffocating hematoma (0,8%) that is similar with international reviews that shows (0,9%).Mortality: 1 patient (0,17%) because of a suffocating hematoma with a Graves disease, hypertension and chronic obstructive pulmonary disease.

Conclusion

Our review,814 cases, shows a prevalence of benign pathology in women. The most common malignant tumor is the Papillary. Compared to the international literature, we observed a higher aggressiveness of the Papillary carcinoma in our population, considering intra thyroid or extra thyroid dissemination and lymph node metastases. That is the reason why we perform total thyroidectomy in all cases regardless the tumor type or stage.

References

[1] Corino M y col. (2011) Programa Nacional de Bocio Nodular (PRONBONO). Estudio multicéntrico de bocio nodular único palpable. *Rev. Endocrin. y Metab* ;48:149-157.

[2] McGuirt W, Marshall R. (1980) Post irradiation carcinoma in thyroid remnant: follicular variant of papillary thyroid carcinoma. *Head Neck Surg.*;38:36-40.

[3] Gauna Alicia, Novelli José Luis. Hipertiroidismo 1a ed. Rosario, UNR Editora, Universidad Nacional de Rosario. (2008):32;345-357.

[4] Novelli JL. (2010) Tratamiento quirúrgico de las recurrencias locoregionales en el carcinoma papilar. *VII Congreso de FASEN.*

[5] Mazzaferri El. (1987) Papillary thyroid carcinoma: factors influencing prognosis and current therapy. *Semin Oncol;*14:315-32.

[6] Mazzaferri El, Jhiang SM. (1994) Long-term impact of initial surgical and medical therapy on papillary and follicular thyroid cancer. *Am. J. Med.* ;97:418-28.

[7] Kowalski L; Novelli J. (2010) Carcinomapapilar de tiroides. *Ed. UNR. Cap.*. 6, pág. 73-76.

[8] Kowalski Luiz Paulo y Novelli José Luis. (2010) Carcinoma papilar de tiroides. Editorial URN Editora. 1^{0}ed; 19:201-211.

[9] Kowalski Luiz Paulo y Novelli José Luis. (2010) Carcinoma papilar de tiroides. Editorial URN Editora. 1^{0}ed; 19:213-219.

[10] Verburg FA, de Keizer B, Lam MG, et al. (2007) Persistent disease in patients with papillary thyroid carcinoma and lymphnodemotastases after surgery and iodine-131 ablationa. *World J. Surg.* ; 31:2309-14.

[11] Alberti G, Zimmet P, Shaw J, Grundy S. (2011) The IDF consensus worldwide definition of the Metabolic Syndrome. Disponible en http://www.idf.org/webdata/docs/IDF_Meta_def_final.pdf.

[12] Wilhelm S.M., Carter C., Tang L., et al. (2004)Bay 43-9006 exhibits broad spectrum oral antitumor activity and targets the RAF/MEK/ERK pathways and receptor tyrosine kinases involved in tumor progression and angiogenesis. *Cancer Res.;*64:7099-7109.

[13] Executive Summary of The Third Report of The National Cholesterol Education Program (NCEP) (2001). Expert Panel on Detection, Evaluation, And Treatment of High Blood Cholesterol In Adults (Adult Treatment Panel III). JAMA; 285: 2486–97.

[14] Sari R; Balci M; Altunbas H; Karayalcin U. (2003) The effect of body weight and weight loss on thyroid volume and function in obese women. *Clin. Endocrinol.* ;59:258–262..

[15] Malaguarnera R; Frasca F; Garozzo A; Giant F; Pandini G; Vella V; Vigneri R; Belfiore A. (2011) Insulin Receptor Isoforms and Insulin-Like Growth Factor Receptor in Human Follicular Cell Precursors from Papillary Thyroid Cancer and Normal Thyroid. *JCEM* ;96(3):766-774.

[16] Ayturk S; Gursoy A; Kut A; Anil C; Nar A; BascilTutuncu N. (2009) Metabolicsyndrome and its components are associated with increased thyroid volume and nodule prevalence in a mild-to-moderate iodine-deficient area. *Eur. J. Endocrinol.* ;161:599–605.

[17] Li X; Lu S; Miyagi E; Katoh R; Kawaoi A. (1999)Thyrotropin prevents apoptosis by promoting cell adhesion and cell cycle progression in FRTL-5 cells. *Endocrinology* ;140:5962–5970.

[18] Rezzónico J; Rezzónico M; Pusiol E; Pitoia F; Niepomniszcze H. (2009) Increased prevalence of insulina resistance in patients with differentiated thyroid carcinoma. *Metab. Syndr. Relat. Disord* ;7:375-380.

[19] Rezzónico J; Rezzónico M; Pusiol E; Pitoia F, Niepomniszcze H. (2011) MetforminTreatment for Small Thyroid Nodules in Patients withInsulinResistance. *Metab. Syndr. Relat. Disord.* ;9:69-75.

[20] Hawk WA, Hazard JB. (1976) The many appearances of papillary carcinoma of the thyroid. *Cleve. Clin.* Q; 43: 207–216.|PubMed|ISI|ChemPort|

[21] Martín-Pérez E, Larrañaga E, Marrón C, Monje F. (1997) Primary papillary carcinoma arising in a thyroid cyst. Eur. J. Surg.;163:143-5.

[22] Carcangiu ML, Bianchi S. (1989) Diffusesclerosing variant of papillary thyroid carcinoma. Clinicopathologic study of 15 cases. *Am. Sug. Pathol.* ;13:1041-9.

[23] Sheu S.I., Schwertheim S., Worm K., Graabellus F., Werner Schmid K.(2007) Diffuse sclerosing variant of papillarythyroidcarcinoma: lack of BRAF mutation but occurrence of RET/PTC rearrangements. *Modern Pathology*;20:779-787.

[24] Vrabie C., Terzea D., Petrescu A., Wallwe M. (2009) The histopathology analysis of the diffuse sclerosing variant of the papillary carcinoma of the thyroid: a distinctive and rare form. *Romanian Journal of Morphology and Embryology*; 50(4):743-748.

[25] Kim H.S., Han B.K., Shin J.H., Sung C.O., Oh Y.L., Song S.Y. (2010) Papillary thyroid carcinoma of a diffuse sclerosing variant: ustrasonographic monitoring from a normal thyroid gland to mass formation. *Korean J. Radiol.* ;11(5): 579-82.

[26] Rodriguez J. Romero P. Wu H. Durand A. et al. (2010) Carcinoma de Células escamosas de tiroides. A propósito de un caso. *Rev. Arg. Endoc. y Metab.*; 47 versión ISSN 1851-3034.

[27] Wu P.S., Leslie P.J., McLaren K.M., Toft A.D. (1989) Diffuse sclerosing papillary carcinoma of thyroid: a wolf in sheep's' clothing *Clin. Endocrinol.* (Oxf); 3(5):535-540.

[28] Romero A., Meza I. (2010) Carcinoma papilar de tiroides, variante esclerosante difusa: un subtipo histológico de difícil diagnóstico. *Rev. Colomb. Cancerol.*; 14(4): 240-244.

[29] D'Addino JL, Pigni MM, Niepomniszcse H. (2008) Carcinoma mucoepidermoideesclerosante con eosinofilia de la glándula tiroides. Comunicación de caso. *Rev. Arg. Cirug.* ;95:15-17

[30] D'Addino JL, Canteros G et al. (2004) Angiosarcomaepiteliode de tiroides con metástasis en hueso. Comunicación de caso clínico. *Revista Argentina de Endoc. y Metabolismo*;41:214-221.

[31] D'Addino JL, Canteros G, Mayorga H, et al. (2005) Metástasis de carcinoma papilar tipo endometroide de útero en glándula tiroides. *Rev. Cirujano General de la Asociac Mexicana de Cirugía;*27:324-327.

[32] Pardal José L. (2010) Complicaciones de la cirugía Tiroidea. Revista de la Sociedad de Otorrinolaringologia de Castilla y Leon, *Cantabria y La Rioja*; 1(4):1-152.

Index

#

A

B

C

D

E

F

G

H

M

N

O

P

Q

R

S

T

U

V

W

X

Y